FINDING
TAMBRI

SHERRY MEEKS

Finding Tambri

Ibex Street Press, Macon, GA

ISBN 978-0-9968043-0-1

Library of Congress Control Number: 2015917708

In memory of three wonderful women

Maebelle

Betsy

Gail

Tambri

"I'm not drowning. Stop watching me."

Vickie observes me from the doorway, drinking her glass of tea. I scrub the side of her tub, and out of the corner of my eye I see her hand go to her hip.

How can she taste the liquid in her glass with the smell of Comet hanging in the room? Kneeling on the tile floor wearing yellow gloves that make my hands sweat, I look up. "What?" I say.

"As soon as you move your skinny ass, I'm pulling down the shower curtain and washing it," she says.

"Why don't you go clean something else in the meantime? I saw the inside of your refrigerator."

She moves past me, sets her glass sideways in the porcelain sink, the ice and tea spilling out. "You could kill a canary in here." She reaches over with one hand and pushes up the window. "You're supposed to keep it ventilated."

The hot outside air circulates and clears my nose. I pull back from the tub and lean on my heels.

Unhooking the rings, she says, "What did you do last night?"

"Slept like a baby."

"Fine, smartass."

"Tended to the horses and then watched T.V." I shrug one shoulder toward her. "Good enough?"

"Okay," she says. I go back to cleaning the tub, and she releases more hooks. "You think I should bleach this?" she says.

"That's the only way to get rid of that disgusting mold, crappy housekeeper." She play-kicks me in the butt and moves toward the washer outside of the bathroom.

I can hear the lawnmower in the backyard. Benny doesn't do housework.

"Listen, Tambri, Benny and me are going to this party tonight at his work. One of the guys is leaving after twenty years."

"What?" I pretend I can't hear her over the running water of the washing machine and the noise of the lawnmower.

"I said—" she says.

I turn the cold handle to rinse the tub. I say, "What?" and turn the water on higher and laugh.

She peeks around the door. "You could hear me the whole time, couldn't you?" she says, flicking water from her fingers toward me.

I turn the water off. "Okay, what are you doing tonight?"

"We're going to this party. Do you want to go with us?" She looks at the ceiling. "There's a dust web in that corner," she says and points with her chin.

"I'll get it." I stand up and pull my gloves off and toss them toward the web.

"Well?" she says.

"I don't know."

"Yeah, Tambri, you're going. You need to meet some new people."

"Maybe I don't feel like going, Vickie."

I pick up the gloves from where they landed on the floor outside the tub. Sometimes I want to shut myself in my house, but Vickie won't let me do that. I know she gets frustrated with me.

"You have to do something sometime," she says. Her voice softens. Someone else would think she might be about to let it go. I know better.

&

We just picked Benny up from his house, and we're on our way to the party. Vickie came by my house early to make sure I was still going. She pulled a dress out of my closet for me, pressed it, and cleaned up a pair of black pumps I hadn't worn since Sammy's funeral. The day of the funeral was a rainy one, and the heels of my shoes sunk into the ground.

The car's warm, and I can feel my curls wilting. Vickie rolled my hair with curlers she had brought from her house. Normally, I just brush my hair and go, but she was determined. The only time my hair was rolled on a regular basis was when I was a kid and stayed over at my grandmother's house.

My grandmother had these pink sponge curlers she used on my hair. She rolled my wet strands tightly around each curler; I can still hear the click of each plastic clamp. They hurt when I finally went to bed, each clip pressing between my head and the pillow. I ended up pulling most of them out during the night.

I'd stay over at her house, and we'd play cards. She's the one who taught me the rules of rummy. When I was about eight, we sat up one night until about two in the morning, and she showed me how to shuffle the cards.

She was a short round woman, maybe five feet tall, but I always remembered wanting to reach her height. I was probably thirteen when I finally did.

Her house didn't smell of mothballs like my friend Stephanie's grandma's house did or anything old like that. She'd stay up drinking coffee until all hours and slept late, and then she'd get up wide awake and throw open all the windows. "We're letting the night slide out and the day slip in," she'd say.

"Now, you take the cards and split them in two. See, honey?"

I eyed those cards wanting to be as steady handed as her.

"Just feed one after another until they're all stacked again." The slick paper clatter of card against card made my ears twist. She gave me the jokers to put in the spokes of my banana seat bike.

"Okay."

I took the cards and held them to my chest as I cut them in two. I placed them on the side table that we were playing on. The lamp on the table was the only light burning in the room. We sat on the opposite outer edges of the triangle of the yellow hue. The dead quiet and the lateness of the night calmed us. I held the stacks in each palm, squeezing them until they bowed inward toward each other.

"Use your pointing fingers to push the cards onto the table and back together." She took a sip of coffee and sat the cup back on the saucer without making any sound.

I pushed the cards with my fingers and they all fell together in a messy pile. I looked at Grandma; she laughed and I laughed. "That's what happens the first few times you try it. You'll get it though. You trust your old granny, don't you?"

"Yep," I said, still laughing.

"Give me the cards for a second and I'll read them for you."

"What does that mean?" I said, hoping she could read them, whatever it did mean.

"I can tell you what each card means for you, depending on where you divide the deck. It's not real; it's just for fun." She mixed the cards in a different way, holding the stack in one hand and letting them slide in small groups into the other. It was easy for her. The smoothness and steady rhythm drew me in. I leaned my head on one arm on the table and watched as she set the deck in front of my eyes.

"Make three stacks."

I picked up half the cards with my free hand and dropped two sections on the table. "Is that good?" I adjusted my eyes to look up into her face.

"That's fine. All right, let's see what we have." She started quickly running through the cards.

"What are you looking for?" I said in a whisper.

"You." She went through four more cards. "Here you are, queen of clubs. That's you with your dark brown hair. Everything that falls after you is about you. Understand?"

I nodded my head.

"Jack of clubs." She held the card up in front of my face for me to get a closer look at the red and black drawing of the man with the crown and funny mustache. "When you grow up you're going to meet a dark-haired young man." She moved her face closer to me as she said, "A nice looking man."

The next card was a ten of hearts. "Ten for sure, you're going to marry him," she said.

I grinned.

"Queen of spades. Maybe that's your dark-haired old grandma."

"Yeah!"

She went through several more cards. "You're going to travel many roads. Who don't, though?" She cackled when she spoke. "Jack of hearts. You're going to have a red or blonde-haired man in your life, too. Ain't that funny? The boys are going to love you."

"You think so, Grandma?" There was this cute boy named Thomas in the fourth grade, whose hair was kind of a sandy color. I wondered if that counted as red or blonde. Boys were starting to notice me.

"Honey, I know that right now, look at how pretty you are. You know who you take after—don't you?"

"You!" We both cackled. She laid several more cards on the table, mostly kings and jacks.

She looked while she ran her fingers across them from left to right, just like she was reading words in a book. She looked at me without smiling.

"What do they mean? Read them, Grandma."

"Nothing much, honey. You're going to be happy with all these people in your life. It's just silliness anyway."

"Yeah?" I said.

She put the cards back in a pile and slid them into their cardboard box.

"I need to practice shuffling some more. Remember, it was a big mess the first time I tried. I want to learn how to make it look easy like you do."

"You'll get it, Tambri. I'm tired. It's late, and we need to find our beds and get our beauty sleep."

"I really wanted to practice some more." We both stood up, and I dropped my head forward just like kids do when they want their way. She usually didn't fall for this; she'd seen her share of kids and grandkids, and she knew all the games.

She leaned over and found a spot on my head without a curler and kissed it. "You can work on it tomorrow as long as you want. You'll eventually control the cards, instead of them controlling you."

I think about my grandmother as we pull into Livingston's Accounting. Vickie said they cleared out the big conference room for the party. There are people milling around, heading toward the door. Vickie looks back at me.

"Tambri, at least try to have a good time, okay?" she says.

I pretend I don't hear her as I slide out of the car. Benny closes my door behind me, and we all move toward the noise of the party.

There are about eight or nine couples here, and maybe four other people besides me who don't seem to be connected to anyone in some way. The couples are easy to spot. Territories marked by physical contact: hand holding, one arm draped over the shoulder of the other or wrapped around a waist, or my least favorite, one person, usually the woman, feeding her mate a Swedish meatball off of her fork. Daniel and I were probably just as bad before everything broke apart.

Vickie is beside me while Benny says hello to his buddies from work. He just saw them yesterday, but everyone acts like it's been years. Big smiles, pats on the back.

The party atmosphere loosens everyone's behavior, not to mention that it looks like the liquor is plentiful. It's loud, and people laugh with mouths wide open, throwing their heads back, then leaning forward to take another sip of a drink.

I want to go home, but I know I'm stuck here until my ride is ready to go. And that means Vickie.

"Come on, let's don't just stand here." She takes me by the elbow and starts introducing me to everyone around the room.

"This is Benny's boss and his wife."

"Nice to meet you. Thank you for having me at your party."

The wife says, "Any friend of our Benny's is welcome here." She beams at Vickie like she's paid her a huge compliment. Nobody else can see it, but I can tell that Vickie's smile is fixed. The "our Benny" comment did not sit well, and Vickie doesn't really care for the wife. According to Vickie, the wife thinks she runs the place and sometimes she'll stop by and check on everyone.

I told Vickie not to let it bother her, and to just imagine kicking the old woman in the ass. She laughed at that. Just talking about kicking the woman in the ass made her feel better.

I meet one more couple, and Vickie seems to like them. She's laughing and smiling, and it's real. Here comes one of the single people, a guy probably around twenty-eight or thirty. He's okay looking, holding a bottled beer in his hand, smiling the entire walk up to our group. Eager.

"Hey, Brad," Vickie says to the guy and hugs his neck. The couple drifts out of our space, and they move on to another conversation.

"Hey, Vick," he says and makes a bear sound as he squeezes her shoulders. They pull apart from the hug, and they look at me.

What? I think.

"This is my friend Tambri," Vickie says looking at Brad, touching her hand to my arm. "This is my friend Brad," she says looking at me. She is smiling like I've never seen her smile before.

"Hello, Brad," I say, and he shakes my hand.

"It's nice to meet you, Tambri. Vickie's given you rave reviews."

Oh, shit. That's what this is about, and that's why I have these curls in my hair.

Vickie turns to Brad looking him right in the face, ignoring me. If I get an opportunity during the party where no one can see me, I'm kicking her right in the shin.

I don't want any of this.

"What did she tell you?" I say. I am trying my best to pull myself together, but I wasn't expecting this. I'm shaky, you know, like when someone comes up behind you and scares you. Just at the moment you're most surprised, the most frightened, you get this sick feeling inside your stomach. I am surprised and nauseous.

"Well, she told me you were pretty, but she lied."

Vickie and I wait for the next thing we know he's going to say.

"You're beautiful."

I laugh and Vickie starts walking away. I'm not letting her get away from me.

"Excuse me, Brad."

"Sure."

I move quickly to catch Vickie; she's trying her best to leave me to flounder with Brad. I grab her by the elbow and yank her back to me.

"What the hell, Vickie?" I say, whispering directly into her ear.

She pushes my fingers off of her arm. "You need this, Tambri."

"What exactly do I need?" I say in a voice that is so low that she probably can't hear me, but she knows what I'm saying.

"You need to get out and meet people."

"I don't want to meet anyone, Vickie. Not anyone."

"Brad is a decent man."

"I can't believe you." I look across the room at Brad, and I can tell he is what Vickie says he is. A decent man. I used to be married to one.

"Tambri, you haven't been out with anyone since you and Daniel divorced."

"I know that, Vickie." I'm about to go on a tear or start crying or both, and she can see it.

"So, it's not good for you," she says in her sweetest tone. The change in her voice makes me remember where we are and I close my eyes, feeling my breath in my chest.

I open my eyes and we look at each other without saying anything, and she knows I've surrendered. She knew that I would in front of Benny's boss and coworkers.

I'm here for the next hour, or two, or however long Vickie feels I need to stay. Apparently, she's the judge at this thing, and she tells me how much time to put in. We stare at each other, one waiting for the other to do something.

"I'm going to get a drink," I say, and leave her standing like an idiot by herself.

I walk to the open bar. "Vodka and pineapple juice," I say, and here comes Brad heading this way. He's a lanky guy, maybe six foot three.

"Hi, again."

"Hi, Brad."

I should ignore him, but I can't. This is Vickie's fault.

"How long have you worked here, Brad?"

"I don't work here. Vickie cuts my hair, and she invited me to the party."

She brought him here just to talk to me? He isn't just some guy that she thought was cute that works with Benny?

Oh, my God.

I gulp my drink. It burns my throat, and the heat slows me down. I drink again and set the glass on the bar. The ice doesn't stand a chance in this room that seems to be getting warmer. I stir my drink with a thin red straw, and I glance at Brad.

"Vickie did a good job on your hair," I say.

He scratches his head, turning red in the face.

"What do you do?" I say.

"I'm in tech support at Harlin's Grocery."

"I shop at the one on Sergeant Street. Do you work at that one?"

"No, but I know the one you're talking about. I work out of the main office. It's about forty-five minutes from here. I make the drive every day."

"I shop there." I know I've said that, but like I said, I'm a little off balance.

"Good," he says, "job security for me." He laughs loudly at his joke. It's not funny, but I can't let him laugh by himself. I smile up at him. It's all I've got to offer.

Vickie is watching from across the room, standing next to Benny. I'm sure he's unaware of this whole thing. I cut my eyes at her, and in response she picks up a cracker, puts a piece of square orange cheese on it, and sticks it in Benny's mouth. She knows how I hate that. I turn back toward Brad.

"What should we do, Tambri?" Brad says.

"What do you mean?" I say taking another sip. I know this won't be the end for Vickie; she's on a mission now.

"Should we talk and get to know each other?"

That was straightforward. I've got to give Brad that. The man doesn't waste any time with words. I scan the room to see who else has come in. Close to Vickie stands a man holding his little girl. Apparently, he and his wife weren't able to find anyone to babysit. The child leans her head on her daddy's shoulder, fighting sleep by crying. The mother stands beside both of them, answering the girl's whimpers with soothing shushes.

"Isn't that sweet? The little girl is adorable," Brad says trying to keep the conversation going. Poor Brad, going in the wrong direction.

"Yes, she is," I say. But, I don't want any more kids. This is information that I know Brad won't want to hear. Losing one was enough, and I will not go through that again. Nope, sure won't.

Brad watches as the little girl finally falls asleep, her daddy rocking his body back and forth to calm her. Brad wants that, it's obvious, being the decent, straightforward kind of guy that he is. He's hoping this setup might turn into something more, and our little girl will have my eyes. I'm so sorry, Brad. I've already had that, and I don't deserve it again.

I swallow the rest of my drink and decide it's time to leave Brad behind.

"Where are you going?" he says.

I'm not really sure. I could go hide out in the ladies room for a while, but I have no doubt that Brad would just stand outside the door waiting. That's not a bad thing, but it's not the thing for me anymore.

"Tambri, where are you going?" he says. My name is becoming too familiar on his lips. Maybe I should set him straight, so he won't think there's anything wrong with him.

"I don't think I'm going anywhere anymore," I say, laughing a little.

"Well, come back over here then," he says, laughing the same way that I did. He's taken the laugh as a sign to become bolder, to flirt a little more.

I walk towards him and make a decision.

"Brad, I'm messed up," I say.

"Well, you do look a little tipsy, but I wouldn't say you're messed up." He reaches forward like he wants to balance me. I pull away before he can make any contact.

"That's not what I mean."

"Then what do you mean?" he says, giving me a big fat grin.

"I'm really messed up. In everyday life, day and night, messed up. Stuff has happened that I don't think I'll ever come back from." I move closer to Brad and pat him on the chest. "I don't deserve someone like you anymore, Brad."

"I'm sorry about all that," he says, and he can't look at me now. He already knows; Vickie's told him. What did she tell him? How did she tell him?

"Tambri, I have no idea what that's like."

It's like your son dying, and you know that you will never recover. You will never be good enough for this world again.

He's still talking.

"But, it doesn't mean that you can't go out and have some fun and see what happens. Everybody deserves that."

I'm staring at him. Not believing this. I'm staring at this man with the horrible haircut, who thinks he knows something about me; I'm staring at him, and I'm trying to figure out who the hell this weirdo thinks he is.

I've been looking at him for a long time now, because he's finally shut up, and he's shifting his weight from one foot to the other. He reminds me of those pink flamingos that you see in Florida. I want to slap him. Slap him as hard as I can.

"I'm going to the little girl's room," I say, walking away from him.

I'm not going to the bathroom. I'm headed toward this group of three people. One of the men is the opposite of Brad, total opposite. He's been watching me on and off all night, and I haven't seen him glance once at the couple holding the kid. Kids are the furthest things from this guy's mind.

Cut

I can't do enough for Tambri, not enough to help her through this. We clean each other's houses on Saturday, and each time we leave her house, and she's locking the door, it's all I can do not to take a water hose to the dingy white wood and red brick of the outside. I stare at the vines that run up and down, and I stop myself from climbing the drainpipe to strip the roped plants that cling to window screens, blocking the light.

I stand still every time, and watch as Tambri walks away from the house that is always empty, except for her. As thin as she's become, there's not much of her there either.

I work at Vivian's Salon on Brookhaven. Vivian doesn't really work there anymore. She's in her seventies, and she can't stand on her feet as long as she needs to. She'll come by once in a while and talk and see how everyone is doing. She always asks about Tambri.

"How's your friend?" she'll say.

"She's okay. You know, it's rough."

"Yeah, it's not fair, is it?" she'll say, running her red-polished fingernails through her blue strands. She cranes her neck like a pelican checking the sagging skin in the mirror.

"It's damn unfair," I'll say. She hugs me, and her jewelry clangs as she walks out the door, her perfume scent lingering behind.

There is no sound to Tambri as she walks, and she doesn't leave anything of herself when she goes away now. She seems to want to disappear.

I'm rolling Mrs. Roberts hair right now. I said I wouldn't deal with this old woman again. Here I am winding another section of coarse gray hair around a green roller. She's always cranky, never happy with what I do, even though she only wants me to work on her hair, and she tips me a dollar every time. A dollar.

"Don't forget, I don't want you using those tiny blue rollers in my hair this time," she says and turns the page of some old magazine. She always picks up the same one. It's her way of ignoring me.

"I'm not. I locked those away before your appointment," I say and laugh.

"Just see that you don't. My hair was so tight and dry last time that I couldn't do anything with it for a week and a half."

Dry just like her ass. I've got better things to worry about than this woman's sorry hair. I know it by the texture. She's always had bad hair, and me using or not using blue curlers isn't going to help or hurt matters.

Mrs. Roberts doesn't talk to me unless she's discussing her hair. I'm a paid servant as far as her thinking goes. Today, I want to talk and to stop thinking about Tambri for just a few minutes. It seems wrong for me to want a break from this. Tambri's not getting one.

It's only me and one other girl, Daphne, working today, and she's just started on a cut and color on Josephine Waters. It'll take Daphne at least two hours to finish her. Josephine's hair is long and thick. It runs below her bra strap. She gets It colored too dark. I think someone mentioned to her one time that she looked like Priscilla Presley, and she took it to heart. The color makes her look older than her thirty-seven years.

"Why don't you let me color your hair, Mrs. Roberts? It'd be beautiful in a shade of ash brown. Chestnut number twelve would work so well with your complexion." I point with another green curler to the chart propped against my mirror.

"I've told you before that I don't want any color. If God wants my hair to be solid white, so be it."

I want to yell at the witch, "What's the difference to God between a perm and hair coloring? He doesn't mind if you curl your hair, but he does get ticked if you color it?"

I'd be damned if this woman isn't insane.

I like what I do, not at this particular moment, but usually I like it. I'm the best at coloring and highlighting. I only use foils when I highlight. I've had some women come in and beg me to pull their hair through a cap of tiny holes.

"It doesn't have to hurt," I tell them. Each and every one is scared of trying something different, even with me being an experienced hairdresser. I can see it in the way they look at me.

It's got to hurt, doesn't it?

Who came up with this anyway? Women have to suffer to look good, to feel good. You won't see a man suffering to look better for a woman. A man is in and out with a fresh haircut in five minutes.

I use the foils on my customers, and they are turned around in their thinking. They can't believe it.

"I love it," they say. I flip the cape off of them and they feel like new. They give me big tips for making them look good without pain. I wish I could figure out how to do that for Tambri.

I did Tambri's hair for her wedding. I'd just graduated from Habersham Technical College. It was just a cut, not a color. Tambri's hair is close to cinnamon number three, brown with just a little bit of auburn highlights.

"Are you okay with me practicing on you?" I asked her as she sat on her closed toilet seat in her bathroom.

"Vickie, just cut it," she said. I was twenty-two and she was twenty. She's always been good about pushing me to do things, supporting me.

Plainly put, I was jealous of her. It seems ridiculous now. Not that she's any less pretty than she was then; it's just that now none of it seems worth worrying about.

"Do you like it?" I asked her when I finished with the cut.

"Vickie, it looks great," she said moving her head from side to side, judging it from all angles in the mirror.

She couldn't see the back, of course, and I didn't offer her a hand mirror. A small gap rested in the upper middle of her hair. My scissors slipped and I cut one section way too short. I think I was nervous about cutting her hair.

I remember thinking a small bird would enjoy sitting in that spot. I hope I didn't do it on purpose. I do wonder about the Freud crap and all. There are no accidents or coincidences, or something like that.

"I can get one of the other girls to redo it. Maybe make it look even better," I said begging.

"Stop," she said.

What was I jealous of? She's always been so pretty and slender, unlike yours truly. I'm not fat, but I'm one of those girls that always weighs just a little more than she should. I've been to Tambri's house before she's gotten up, and she'll come to the door half-asleep, and she looks nothing like I do. Any man would be happy to wake up next to her.

And the thing that bothered me the most was that she was about to get married to a good-looking and kind man, and I wasn't married, yet.

"Are we still going to celebrate your twenty-first birthday?" I said, trying not to stare at the back of her head.

"You know we are." She patted me on the arm. "Help me try on my dress," she said as she walked toward her bedroom.

"Again?" I said.

"Yes, it's fun, and you can try on your bridesmaid dress."

I didn't really want to try it on, but I couldn't tell her no.

I put the thing on. Tambri had done her best for me. It didn't look bad, but it bunched in the middle, around my thick waist.

"Vickie, I knew that blue would go good with your eyes."
My dress was a teal blue with tiny silver threads running
through it. It was tea length, stopping just below my knees.
I still have it in the back of my closet.

But she looked so much better standing in front of that
mirror. I kept telling myself that she was supposed to look
the best; it was her wedding after all.

"You look so pretty," she said putting her arm around my
shoulder and squeezing.

She always means the things she says about me. I've always
wondered how someone so pretty can be so nice.

"What are you doing?" Mrs. Roberts says.

I got the tiniest spot of neutralizer on the very top of her
forehead. She's flailing her hands around her eyes like some
got in there. She's grabbing tissues, wiping her eyes, then
her forehead, and wrinkling her already wrinkled nose at
the smell.

I'll be damned if this woman isn't ridiculous.

It doesn't matter how old people get; they are children.
Mrs. Roberts has got to be close to eighty, but I know without asking anybody that this is the way she's always been.
Complaining when she was little when some boy she liked
threw dirt too close to her face. People are children. They
just drive cars, have jobs, and make babies.

Tambri's baby was beautiful. She got pregnant three months
after she got married. Her husband Daniel, ex-husband now,
named him Samuel. We called him Sammy. There was no
doubt that baby belonged to them. He had green eyes like
Tambri and blonde hair like Daniel. He was into all kinds
of things, just like little boys are.

It almost killed Tambri when Sammy died. He was four years old. It almost killed me, but I held it in as much as I could around her. Still do. It wouldn't be helpful to anybody if I said anything.

I can see Tambri crossing the street in her work clothes. She's wearing her navy pants and smock. People would think she was seventeen or eighteen in that getup, and she's twenty-six. She looks like a kid, but she doesn't act like a kid that much anymore. She's not paying attention to the traffic, being careless not watching the cars. That's when she acts like a kid, when she doesn't care what happens to her.

She's started this thing with going out with men. Sounds silly when I say it that way. She hadn't gone out for the longest, and then it was like she flipped some kind of switch. It's the type of men that she's picking. Most of them are just a little left of what she used to go for, some way far to the left.

Of course, Daniel was her first true boyfriend. So, maybe I'm wrong and she just got lucky with Daniel. This thought of her purposely picking these men keeps sticking in my brain, but there isn't a damned thing I can do about it. And still, I'm not sure if what I'm sensing is even real. Since Sammy died, I haven't felt quite right, either.

"Are you done, yet?" Mrs. Roberts says. She's only saying that because she saw me stop for a second to watch Tambri.

I put the plastic cap on her head and hand her another magazine.

"Twenty-five minutes, Mrs. Roberts."

Tambri comes through the door and leans on the counter.

"Hey, Vickie," she says, trying to smile. "Hey, Mrs. Roberts."

Mrs. Roberts nods to Tambri. Tambri looks at me as if she wants to say, "I thought you were done with her."

I shrug my shoulders.

"Vickie, do you have a few minutes to trim my hair?"

"Yep, Mrs. Roberts has a little while with the neutralizer."

"I'm not going to wait for you to finish Tambri's haircut," Mrs. Roberts says. "You better be done with her by the time this perm stuff is finished."

We both walk past my station to Regina's. Regina went to Savannah for a few days with her new boyfriend. He's no good, but you can't tell anybody anything.

I would normally put my client in another chair while I was waiting on the neutralizer to finish. I know better than to ask Mrs. Roberts that. She'd throw the biggest fit.

Tambri sits down in the chair without saying much, and I can tell she's trying to avoid looking in the mirror at herself. She's got shadows under her eyes. I turn her away from the mirror and start combing through her hair.

"How long has it been since I've cut your hair?"

"A couple of months, maybe?"

"I've told you that you can't wait that long. You've got split ends all over the place."

"Split-end this," she says, and she shoots a bird into the mirror and we both laugh.

Sammy died right after I married Benny. Tambri was at the house a lot more than usual after that, and Daniel didn't come by much at all. I think he wanted to be by himself. Benny stayed out of Tambri's and my way. Benny's not a big talker. I make up for that, but for that time he talked even less. He seemed like a ghost in our house moving through only to pass from one room to the next. Or, maybe Tambri and me were the ghosts, floating around in some strange place where children die.

If I could give her anything to make her feel better, I would, from driving her to work, to fixing her dinner, to offering her a place to stay in the guest bedroom.

"I still have a husband to sleep with at home, you know," she said to me. This was before things went bad with their marriage. They were already drifting apart in their grief. I can see that now.

"Yeah," I said trying to laugh. It was too much for them. It wasn't that they didn't love each other, they did. It's just that they couldn't watch each other in that kind of shape.

"You can't fix this, you know," Benny said one night while he was reading a book. He was lying next to me in our bed, and his voice made me jump. The sound of it pulled me back to where he was.

"Fix what?"

"What's going on with Tambri," he said, and that was all he said.

Yeah, but I can comfort the hell out of her and watch out for her. I owe her that.

Her hair is like silk as I comb it. It's the only thing that shines on her now. She bites her nails down to nothing, and her hands are rough from the horses. I want to give her a manicure, but she always says no. She doesn't want anything that might make her feel good.

I brush and brush her hair.

"Vickie, are you going for the hundred strokes?" Tambri says.

"What if I am? I'm the hairdresser. You're only the client."

"Uh-huh," she says. I can only see the side of her face in the mirror, but I can tell she's smiling a little.

"You know this really needs to be washed."

"I don't have time."

"Why, where are you going? Home, to sit in front of the T.V.?"

"I need to take care of the horses."

"Tambri, it will take all of three minutes for me to wash your hair." I pull her up by her shoulders while I'm talking. I don't want to give her too much time to think about it. She walks over to the sink and sits down in front of one and lays her head back in slow motion, almost like she's waiting for a blade to strike her neck. I blink, not liking the thought, and reach for the shampoo.

I wash her hair and then use a deep conditioner. She doesn't really need the conditioner, but a lot of my ladies say that it's soothing when I put the conditioner in and massage their scalp with the warm water. I use apple flavor on Tambri's hair. It's quiet except for Daphne's scissors and the sound of the water coming out of the sprayer as I move it around in circles on Tambri's head. She seems relaxed with her eyes closed, and the lines in her forehead ease.

"I have to take care of the horses before my date tonight," she says in a soft tone.

"Who are you going out with?" I say in the same volume, not wanting to spoil the stillness. That's another thing; she doesn't really tell me about these guys.

"That guy that works at UPS. He came in here one time."

"I think I know who you're talking about. Kind of a burly guy, needs to do a few pushups?"

"Well, I guess that's one way to describe him," Tambri says, and she laughs. "I think he looks like he's in good shape. He's just a big guy."

A big jackass, I want to say, but I don't. He's a smart ass, who thinks he knows everything, and who thinks he looks ten times better than he actually does. Before all this, Tambri and me would have made fun of a guy like that. There were guys like that in high school.

"It has been twenty-one minutes!" Mrs. Roberts says yelling as loud as she can with her scratchy old-lady voice. Tambri jumps up straight to her feet. I know that if I were right beside Mrs. Roberts this minute, I would beat her.

"Tambri, sit back down. You still have conditioner in your hair."

She sits back, and she seems dazed. There's no telling the last time she's slept.

"Put your head back, honey," I say to her, and she obeys.

"Twenty-two minutes!" The noise of the woman goes all through me. I want to tell her to shut up. And I might do it if it were just me and Tambri in here. I can tell Daphne and Josephine are trying hard not to listen, or maybe to listen.

"Is it all out?" Tambri says, opening her eyes looking at me upside-down from the sink bowl.

"Yeah, it's all out."

"Listen, I'd better get home."

"Your hair is soaking wet. It'll only take me a couple of minutes to cut it."

"That's okay. Thanks for shampooing it, Vickie." I wrap a towel around her head as she rushes to the door.

"I'll come by later and finish it for you at your house," I say.

"No, Vickie, you can't. I have a date remember?"

I shake my head like I'm saying, "Oh, yeah, I forgot." I didn't forget. I was just hoping she would.

She smiles and slips out, fading into the orange evening.

I turn to Mrs. Roberts and give her the glare of her lifetime. She looks at me likes she's going to say something and then changes her mind. Her mouth's still open as she turns her eyes back to her book and away from me.

I take her to the sink and rinse her hair out as rough and as quick as I can.

"What is wrong with you?" she says in a kind of scared voice. She's trying to stay strong, but she's got no backbone. No deep conditioner for her.

"Go back to the chair, Mrs. Roberts."

"Stop ordering me, Vickie. You know this will affect your tip."

"Keep the dollar," I say in a tone that startles me a little. She opens her mouth to say something, but thinks better of it and flaps it back shut.

One roller after another I yank from her hair.

"Ow!" she says, and tries to turn around to look at me in the face, especially since I won't look at her reflection in the mirror. I comb the rat's nest out. No touching up with the curling iron. No hairspray.

We walk to the cash register, and she places her money on the glass counter. She always pays in cash, too old to use any kind of card.

"Mrs. Roberts, I won't be able to do your hair anymore," I say to her. I'm not really looking at her; I'm looking above her head at the beige wall behind her.

"What?" she says. "You always do my hair."

"Not anymore."

She's stunned as she adjusts the bag on her arm and walks out.

"Keep the change," she says as the door closes and the bell rings behind her. I glance down at the wadded money, counting. A dollar tip.

Forty-Nine Percent

They've got the air going, and the coolness draws me and my buddy Mike in, as I glide past the slot machines with the flashing red and green lights that glitter and rotate, enticing me to play. The place calls to me with everything so shiny and bright, just like Tambri.

"You want to look around, man?" Mike says.

"Sounds good," I say as we walk in different directions. My clammy hands are limp in my jean pockets; so much is riding on this for me and Tambri. We're going to be married in a couple of weeks, and I want to start things the way they should be. I really don't want to hurt her.

"Drink, sir?" A waitress says to me.

"No, thanks," I say. I'm not sure how much the drinks are, or how much to tip. I watch the waitress disappear into a crowd of people wishing I'd ordered something to calm my nerves.

All the people that work here wear white shirts, tucked into black straight pants like tuxedos. Everyone's dressed the same except the cocktail waitresses; they wear white shirts that are cut low in the front with little puffy sleeves for the arms. I think my first wife had a blouse like the waitresses, peasant blouses. My first wife's shirt wasn't low cut. I don't think it's good for a man's wife to dress that way.

Mike's the one who came up with the idea to go gambling before the wedding. A guy who used to work with me named Bennett Sampson threw a party about a month ago. Bennett's wife Sandra is from New Orleans, and I think she misses it. Especially during Mardi Gras, now that she lives in Georgia. So, every year they have a few of us over, and we drink beer and have crawfish, boiled potatoes, corn on the cob, and the cake with the little plastic baby in it.

It was on a Friday, and I got there before Tambri did. I was ready to get things going, and I went straight from work to Bennett's.

There was a bonfire in the backyard, and all the men were sitting or standing around, while the women and the kids were inside in the kitchen. Once in a while Bennett's three-year-old son, Brice, would run outside and circle the fire. His mother didn't want him outside running around.

"Bennett, make him come in," she'd say yelling to her husband. He'd pick Brice up by the armpits and tote him back inside.

I was sitting closest to the fire, a little below everybody else, in this short lawn chair that belonged to Sandra. Once in a while I'd pick up a pinecone and toss it in the blaze. All the other guys, Bennett, Mike Stroud and the Gardner brothers, Travis and Deck, would watch as the fire would spark more and listen to the noise from the little cone burning down to nothing.

Nobody was in a hurry, and we drank the cold beer. The heat and smell of burning wood, and the movement of the fire held us there, and we faced it with our backs to the cold.

Mike talked about wanting to go on a road trip. It was just an excuse to get away from his wife because they're always arguing. I understand. With me and my first wife, we were fighting and arguing just about every day and most nights. I'm sad things got out of hand sometimes. I want things to be different between me and Tambri. I really don't want to hurt her.

But, it's not that easy sometimes. Is it? You're sitting there watching the game with a score of thirteen to fifteen, and your wife just won't let up. Won't let up at all.

I think about how it's going to be with Tambri and me. Sometimes, I think about it so much, it feels like it's a dream that I keep having. It has to be good this time.

"I've been wanting to go gambling somewhere. I haven't been in a while," Mike kept saying.

"Like where?" I said, finally giving in and saying what he wanted somebody to say.

"I've been to Tunica, Mississippi a couple of times."

"Yeah?" Deck said while he walked to Mike's truck, pulling his fourth beer from the cooler in the back. "This lady that Michelle knows said a friend of hers won forty-five thousand dollars there on the triple-seven machine." He took a long sip of his beer. "I'd like to go."

There is no way that his wife, Michelle, would ever let him go anywhere without her. She's always trying to keep a handle on his drinking, but it doesn't seem to do her any good.

I ignored Deck while Mike continued to push for Tunica.

"Yeah," said Mike. He was already planning the trip in his head. I could tell. Mike was Mike and he was going to do whatever he wanted to do.

"We need to go, especially you," Mike said pointing to me with the bottom of his can of Budweiser.

"Why me?" I said laughing.

"You're getting married, you need the money."

About that time, Tambri was at my ear saying, "Hey, Baby."

I didn't see her come up at all; I was too busy listening to Mike. All the guys were looking her over.

"Hey, Baby," I said, and I smiled at all the guys. I never turned my head toward her, and she kissed me on the top of the head. I could hear her walk away, and they watched her all the way to the house. I liked it. And I get to lay my hands on her anytime I want.

She opened the screen door, and Brice busted out again. He ran toward us and said yelling, "Butterfly, butterfly."

We saw what he was pointing to, but it wasn't a butterfly; it was a moth. It was pretty, though. We watched as it circled us and stopped, hanging just above the fire. I guess it was attracted to the light.

"Hey, look at that," Deck said as all of us watched, thinking it was pretty.

It flew to me and landed on my hand. I looked it over as it twisted its feelers and walked around on the topside of my hand like it knew me. It had big wings that were striped dark and light green, and it was fatter than a butterfly. It moved to the palm of my hand and I flinched at the feel of it. I realized how weird it was, sitting on my hand.

"That thing likes you, man," Mike said. He was laughing and looking at me.

"Oh, yeah?" I said. I thumbed at it hard, until I made contact and it flew off. I sipped my beer.

"You didn't have to do that," Mike said shaking his head and laughing.

❧

Mike just told me that you get all the free drinks you want as long as you're playing, and I'm going to play a lot. Mike's been teaching me some of the rules of blackjack, and I'm going to put them to good use.

When Mike first mentioned about this trip, I thought it was a bad idea, but I've changed my mind. Maybe this is the way to keep things straight in our marriage. I really don't want to hurt Tambri.

She's been hurt enough with her child dying and everything.

With me and my first wife, most of the arguments started because of money. One time both our cars broke down within two days of each other. Mine was a busted radiator, and her car fell apart because she didn't mention the oil light had come on. That fight lasted even after both cars were fixed.

I'm excited about being here. Someone has to win and if Tambri and me can start this thing out with enough money to keep things running smooth—God, it could be so sweet. All I want is to have Tambri and live like normal people do.

I met Tambri when I went to Dr. Kimberly's office to work on the copier. The machine was in the hallway, just outside the room where Tambri drew the blood, just in sight distance of where she stood most of the time. The copier was making a black line on every copy that printed. Imagine a little black line bringing two people together. I am lucky.

It was raining that day, and I dripped water on the floor as I walked down the hallway. Donna, the receptionist yelled after me, "Be careful, people have tracked most of the afternoon."

I ran the machine a couple of times and saw the line for myself. I tried cleaning the glass first, but that didn't help anything. I looked up as I was letting the lid of the copier back down, and there Tambri was in her white little room. She was a light in the middle of that colorless space.

She wore a purple smock with green dinosaurs on it, and purple pants. She was a flower with her dark hair and green eyes.

I remember thinking that I wished I had worn my button down shirt and my jeans. Not my damned work shirt with my name embroidered on it. I felt like I was about six.

She pulled white doctor's gloves off her hands, and realized I was there. She wasn't surprised to see me. I'm guessing she knew I was going to be there, sooner or later. She'd probably been listening to the complaints of her coworkers every time they made copies.

"Hey, I'm here to fix the copier," I said to her from the hallway talking way too loud.

"Hope you can fix it," she said as she threw her gloves in a small white garbage can.

"I'll do my best," I said, as I searched in my bag to see what tool might fix the thing, but I hadn't even really looked inside the copier yet. I was having problems concentrating on my work when I was trying to think of something else to say to her.

"Nice smock," I said, and I tried to laugh a little to let her know I was kidding.

"I only wear it when everything else is dirty," she said and laughed with me.

There was really nothing else to say, and it only took me five minutes to realize the problem with the copier was the drum.

"I have to order the part; I should have it in the next few days," I said.

"Thanks," she said as I slid up the hallway and back out into the rain.

I went back the Friday of that week. I had the part the day before, but I wanted to time it for Friday, late in the day. I swung by my house and changed into jeans and my burgundy shirt first.

She had her back to me in her little room when I started working on the copier. She was drawing blood from a lady that had to be at least eighty-five years old. I don't know if Tambri knew I was standing there or not, but she didn't say anything to me until she finished with the lady.

"Are you feeling alright, Mrs. Pennell?"

"I'm fine," the lady said. She looked a little shaky, not from the blood and all, just from being old.

"Okay, let me help you up."

Tambri faced her, and pulled the lady up holding her under the elbows. Tambri wasn't much bigger herself, but you could tell she was use to lifting dead weight. She patted the taped gauze on the lady's arm and said, "Now, leave that on your arm for at least an hour. It will bruise less if you do."

"Thank you, sweetheart."

"You're welcome. Is there someone out front waiting for you?"

"My grandson, you should meet him."

"Hey, Tambri," I said. "If you want I can help her to the front."

Tambri turned around and looked at me. She knew I was there all the time because she wasn't surprised, again. She looked at my shirt and smiled at me like she was saying hello without saying it.

"No, I can make it myself," the lady said. She said thank you to Tambri again and made her way up the hallway moving slowly, using her umbrella as a cane.

"Hello, Mr. Copier Repairman," Tambri said. She was in a playful mood, just like I knew she would be late on a Friday.

"Hey, I have the part. It shouldn't take me long to replace the old one."

"You always bring the rain with you," she said. She was being friendly, and that was good. I made sure not to push things.

She was watching me like she was looking for something.

"It did rain the last time I was here, didn't it?"

"Yep, and now it's going to rain, again. And here you are."

"I'll try for snow, next time." She laughed and looked at me sideways and then lowered her eyes. She walked back to her counter, wrote the old lady's name on a sticker and put it on the vial.

"You were really good with that lady," I said, stepping into her room.

"Well, she's in here every few months. It hurts me when the older people come back after I've taken blood. They always bruise in blue and purple, just like beat-up fruit."

"Yeah," I said. I could tell the thought of that made her sad, and I moved away from it. "Well, I guess I better do what I came to do."

I turned my back to her and walked back out to the hall-way, squatted down and opened the front door of the copier. I listened as she made noise moving around her room. I could feel the shift in the air as she walked across it, putting the vial in a small refrigerator. I glanced at her without her seeing, still moving my hands inside the machine like I was working hard.

She moved differently, adjusting her hair, pulling the one clip that was holding everything in place from the back of her head, smoothing the hair away from her face with her lean fingers, clenching the clip between her teeth, securing all the strands more neatly, her face flushed in pink.

I turned back to my work when she would have caught me. "I'm changing the toner, too."

"Okay," she said.

I finished with the machine and closed the door. Black powder covered my hands and I stood up, looking for the sink. She was watching me. "It's over here," she said as she moved to the left of the sink. She turned on the water for me.

"Soap and water," she said.

She folded her arms in front of her and leaned her backside against the counter.

"Thank you, kindly," I said, walking towards the sink. All I wanted to do was look at her. She was close when I reached the sink and before I washed my hands, I pulled my first two fingers across the inside crease of her arm, transferring black toner to her skin. I could see through to her pale blue veins.

"I've marked you," I said.

"Watch that, now," she said and laughed.

"Now you know how your patients feel."

"Yeah, or an abused peach." She laughed and brushed the toner from her arm.

She was quiet as the water poured over my hands, and splashed onto the stainless steel of the sink. Both of us listening as Donna said goodbye to the last patient. "See you at your next appointment, Mr. Simmons." We heard her lock the door.

I dried my hands. "I'm going out with a couple of my buddies tonight." I said it real low, where Tambri almost couldn't hear me. She strained to hear, but she understood what I was saying.

"Where?"

"We're going to that new bar on Francis Street."

"Burton's?"

"That's it. Have you been there?"

"No, but my best friend is always talking about wanting to go."

She didn't want to meet me alone, and I was thinking that was a good thing. Shows what kind of woman she is.

"The two of you should meet us there tonight."

She went quiet for a minute, thinking. I remember I reached for another paper towel, like my hands were still wet. But that wasn't it; I just couldn't stand her not saying anything.

"What time do you think?"

She had already made up her mind about me.

❧

Mike is checking out a $5 blackjack table. I want him to go first, so that I can watch. I want to get the feel of it.

Mike sits down and says hello to everyone at the table. He's in the third seat from the left, and he wants to sit in the first seat because that's the big shot seat. Another man sits there with his red-headed wife next to him. She's cute, about thirty-three, and Mike keeps flirting with her. He's crazy with her husband sitting right there; nobody seems to mind and everyone's in a good mood. All the great noise, and lights, and drinks flowing, he doesn't even have to move from his seat; the waitresses in the short skirts come by and take orders. Mike tips them one of his smaller chips, maybe a dollar or two. He is so smooth and if his wife knew how he acted—she'd have a fit.

He plays three hands and wins all three. This hand is his fourth. The dealer gets blackjack on the first try which means that everyone loses, unless Mike's got blackjack, too.

"Even money," Mike says before the dealer looks in his mirror to see what he has. Mike likes to push things. He didn't take even money, so he had to push.

I hate being pushed. It doesn't mean anything. You don't win and you don't lose, him sitting there with blackjack and not winning anything.

But everybody seems happy, and I want to be part of the group. Two other people sit down on the right side of the table, and that leaves a spot for me beside Mike. I move in, and the dealer moves to another table. The new guy is about fifty-five with a belly that strains the buttons on his shirt.

"Checking in," he says to the pit boss. The dealer takes my $100 and exchanges it for twenty $5 chips. It's hard to believe those little chips represent money when they look like something from Monopoly.

I'm sweating sitting here. I put down a $5 bet to start, and my first card is a jack of clubs. The dealer makes his second pass with the cards and mine is an eight. I need to stay.

These are good cards, and I'm twisting my ankles and moving my feet, trying to keep the nervousness out of my hands. The dealer gets a four, and the dealer's other card is turned down. I run through Mike's explanation of the game in my mind. A four is good. The house always has to hit on a six or less. I'm hoping he has a ten card under there and he ends up busting on the next card.

Everybody passes on another card as we all think the same thing.

"I know that's a ten card under there," Mike says. He's acting like he's talking to everyone, but he's mostly looking at the redhead.

"You have got to be right," I say. I'm not looking at anybody; I'm watching the cards.

Everybody nods, liking what we're saying. We're all in agreement. The dealer puts down an eight of clubs. Good, good, good. He turns his other card over, and it's a queen of spades.

❧

One hundred-and-forty-one dollars is what I took away from the table last night. Mike said your best odds are at the blackjack table, and that's where I stayed.

When I got back to my room I was keyed up. I looked around my room, pulled the drawers out to see if anyone had left anything inside, and opened the curtains to look at the parking lot five stories below me.

I didn't get much sleep because the bed was hard, the pillows were flat and because so much is riding on this. I had problems with the shower this morning, and I'm planning on talking to somebody at the front desk. The drain plug kept falling in and stopping the water from flowing out, and I had to pull the plug out, sticking my hand into the nasty water three times. By the time I finished, I felt so frustrated that I pulled the shower curtain too hard and ripped it from a few of the rings.

I hit the tables at 7:45 this morning before Mike got up. He says the player has a forty-nine percent chance of winning, while the house has fifty-one percent, and that's what's important about playing blackjack.

I remember what Mike taught me while I play the game alone, tucking the odds alongside my dream of me and Tambri.

Worry Dolls

I pulled the little dolls from my underwear drawer before Vance got home. They're resting in my sweater pocket. I put my hand in my pocket feeling the six stick bodies under my fingers; I twist them changing their order inside my pocket. I walk toward the bedroom to put them back. Vance wouldn't like it if he knew I kept something that my first husband Daniel had given me.

"Where are you going?" Vance says.

Half the time he doesn't pay attention to me. I met Vance one day when I was working at Dr. Kimberly's. He came by to fix the copier for the office, and we got married eight months later. We've been married a year-and-a-half now. A long enough time for the honeymoon to fade and the boxing gloves to come out.

"Nowhere, I guess." I turn toward the kitchen, and he refocuses on Channel Six's news.

"I want mashed potatoes for dinner," he says.

"Okay," I say, just glad that he's not wondering where I was headed.

"Honey, can you get me a glass of milk?" He burps loud and then it turns into a burping song. He laughs between burps, and I can't help but laugh with him.

"I think I had a not-so-great ham sandwich at lunch," he says, laughing and burping in between words.

"Where did you get it from?"

"From here, but I forgot to take the cooler, and it sat in the car in the sun most of the morning."

"Are you sure you feel like eating something right now?" I walk into the kitchen for his milk.

"Yeah. Mashed potatoes are supposed to be comfort food. Maybe they'll comfort my stomach."

I walk back in the living room and hand him the glass. "Not that kind of comfort," I say.

"I know that," he says. He glances away from the news and stares me right back into the kitchen.

I sit at the table peeling potatoes. He's changed the channel to the Braves game, and it doesn't sound like they're doing so well.

"You can't keep letting your players get on base and then not make it home," he says at the television. There's not much more to the baseball season. The days are getting shorter, and I see the last light filtered through the blinds. The night starts to settle in as I finish the last potato.

The Braves lose, and he's flipping channels again. I'm pretty sure the burping has calmed down. I dump the potatoes into the water on the stove and turn the burner to high.

When people ask me about my son, people who haven't seen me in a while, I get quiet and they lean forward listening for the secret, and one by one their faces fall like the branches of a sick tree when I say in a whisper, "He died." The women ask without thinking, "What happened?"

It's the natural response. Then, they stop and touch me. The women do, always.

I was in the grocery store on the cereal aisle with a box of Cheerios in my hand when Evelyn Banks squeezed my shoulder with her short fat fingers. She said over and over, "It's all right, Darling."

Marion Cooper wrapped her arms around my waist while we were in the post office (she's a full foot shorter than me). Her embrace strangled me, and she held it there for a full minute while I closed my eyes and listened to the sound of stamping on envelopes and the guy behind the counter saying, "Next."

When they put their hands on me, my stomach caves inward and I ache to slide from their arms and sink to the floor.

It was easy to size Vance up when he walked into my little world at Dr. Kimberly's.

He was trying to cover up what he was; even changing his clothes before the second time he came to see me. The way he held his shoulders way back and his chest forward when he talked to me, I knew him. He even put his hands on me that second day I saw him, marking my arm with black toner. He was spelled out to me, and I took him anyway.

I pull my pocket open and glance down to make sure the contents are still there. They're made out of matchsticks and they're tiny; each not as tall as my thumb with dark faces painted with eyes and skinny bodies covered in bright paper clothes.

They remind me of what it was like before Sammy died. I know there will be no going back. "They'll be no going back," I say to the boiling potatoes.

"What?" Vance says over the television.

"Nothing." He doesn't hear me; he's too involved with whatever he's watching.

Daniel gave me the dolls just a couple of months into our marriage. God, we were happy.

"You worry too much, Tambri," Daniel said and handed me a small white plastic bag that contained the dolls. It was true then, but now I know it does no good, might as well try to not think about anything.

"You're supposed to whisper a worry to each doll and put them under your pillow at night," Daniel said. I poured the dolls onto my lap.

"Then what?" I kissed him on his temple and crossed my arms over his shoulder while we sat on our dark blue couch. I leaned in closer to his face to watch his mouth move, and the dolls watched with me. I was only twenty.

"The worry goes away by the next morning. Gone. Or, so they say." He laughed, embarrassed, talking dolls with me.

"Who's they?" I couldn't help but prod him a little more.

"Mrs. Springhill."

"At the convenience store? I didn't know they started selling those kinds of things."

"I think she does when the owner's not there. She had them tucked under the counter. She pulled them out when I was paying for gas."

"Yeah?" I said waiting for more from him.

"Yep, that's where they came from. I think Mrs. Springhill used to hang out with your fortune-telling grandmother."

"Sounds like," I said.

I'm me, and Vance is not even close to me. Opposite is not really the right word. He doesn't believe the same things I believe. He doesn't like olives or horses, and he doesn't like this bench I have in my living room. It sits by the front door, and he's all the time making remarks about it.

"I don't think I've seen anything uglier than that bench."

He knows my first husband made it, and Vance and I both know that my first husband's not a carpenter. It really isn't the greatest looking thing. It's not even level. I put a rubber ball on it one time just to see it roll to the floor.

Tuesday before last, Vance came in drunk. It isn't an everyday occurrence, but it does happen. He came in and slammed down on the bench with his whole body like he was trying to crash it. The right side of his torso is black and green streaked because of it. You can see exactly where the boards made their marks.

Oak is not forgiving.

"This thing isn't even comfortable," he said.

"It's just to take your shoes off if you want to at the door."

"When do we do that?" he said. His speech was slurred, going from very loud to a whisper. I knew what he was asking. Why do we need this bench that your first husband and dead child sat on? Why do you keep things like this? I thought I would leave it alone and maybe he'd just fall asleep on the damn thing.

He wore grey flip-flops, one dangling between his big toe and longer second toe. "Oh, you mean like these shoes?" And he kicked them straight out in front of him. He was aiming for me, but I can dodge a flying flip-flop.

His eyes were glazed more than usual.

"How much have you been drinking?"

"I don't know. Tommy was buying." I can't stand that Tommy, and Vance knows it. Tommy will fleece anybody out of whatever he thinks he can get.

"What'd you give him for the beers?" I said.

"He wanted a ride to High Falls. Dumb son-of-a-bitch wanted to see the waterfall at night. Who does that? Especially without a woman."

I was wearing a cotton skirt, and he started looking at my legs.

"Did you drive him there?"

"No, he passed out before I could," he said lowering his voice to a whisper. He reached forward and grabbed the hem of my skirt.

"You think you're up to that?" I pushed his hand away and moved back about a foot—just out of his reach. If he wanted to get me, he'd have to at least stand up.

"What do you say we break this bench in right?"

I could see the look coming into his eye. All squinty, pissed at the world because he thinks he's second rate. Well, he's the one that's put himself there.

"You come here," he said trying to look sexy, leaning across the back of the bench.

I didn't say anything, just watched him like he was some kind of insect.

"I mean it," he says.

He was too drunk to do anything, and I said, "I don't feel like it."

He stared at me like I was the insect, looking me up and down.

He stood up fast, and I thought he was coming after me. But he ran back out the front door that he'd left open. I thought he was sick or something. I peeked through the screen door, squinting my eyes to see him in the darkness. I couldn't see him; he was somewhere in the backyard, moving fast, running away. I couldn't hear anything for a few minutes, and I sat on the bench, wondering how much of a lean there was to it. I'd seen the truck parked out front, two wheels on the grass, the other two on the concrete driveway. Wherever he was going, he was going on foot. I've tried to care about him, but he makes it too damned hard.

I sat on the bench, straining my ears to hear something. He was still running in his bare feet, this time toward the house. I stood up, waiting for whatever was coming through the door.

And then he slammed open the screen door with the hedge clippers in his hand.

Was he going to kill me? I stood there, trying to think. Is that what I wanted? He stopped dead in front of me, his irises dilated. If I stood there long enough, he'd make up my mind for me.

"Enough," he said, the lines of his face pulled. He turned to the bench, holding the closed hedge clippers by the wooden handles above his head. He swayed with the heavy tool. His feet were wet, and his own weight brought him down. The clippers fell from his hands and landed on the floor as he dropped forward on top of the bench. He couldn't hold himself there, and he slid even farther down onto the wooden floor beside the clippers. He lay stomach down with the dirty bottoms of his feet facing the ceiling.

My hands were in fists raised in front of my open mouth. I didn't remember moving. His body rose in slow breaths and eased back down to the floor. The tantrum ended.

I knelt next to him and touched his back, rubbing it. He turned his head to me with dirt on his cheek. He touched my arm, and I put my hand into his. For that one moment, I worried about him.

I've felt bad about it since it happened. Maybe it's my fault that he got so upset because I've kept the bench there. When he asked me last weekend about going to a yard sale with him, it made me glad to say yes.

I was in my usual place on my couch trying to fall asleep. It's easier for me to fall asleep with the distraction of the television. But I never stay there; I guess I think I don't deserve any sleep. I get up instead of just lying there. From the couch, to the bathroom, to pulling back the covers, I wake up more with each movement and each light switch that I flip. I put my body in bed and that's it. No sleep.

"You want to go with me in the morning?" he said while I considered going to bed, twisting the ends of my hair in my fingers.

"Where?"

"There's an estate sale in Warner Robins."

An estate sale is a yard sale for a dead person.

"Okay," I said, twisting my hair, thinking about the opportunity to make things up to him.

As he was driving us there the next morning, he looked over, lifting the corner of his mouth, smiling, causing creases in his cheek. It's rare that we're in the same mood at the same time, especially somewhat of a good one. It was early in the morning, and we were probably just sleepy.

"You want some coffee?" I asked as he steered with one hand and looked at the address on the tiny slip of paper he'd scribbled on.

"Hang on, I can't read this." The coffee was probably stale anyway. He gave the paper to me. I can't ever read his writing. I prepared to strain my eyes, and I brought the sheet within reading distance. It looked like 483 or 452 or 782 Greene, Greyer, Books, or maybe Dove Drive, or Road, or Bridge. I turned it upside down.

"I gave it to you the right way." How could he have known that? He couldn't read it.

"782 Greene Road." I took a stab at what it might possibly be.

"Good. They're supposed to have furniture and jewelry there."

"Yeah?"

"Maybe a ring that's worth a lot of money. Or a pretty necklace or a tiara."

I didn't know he knew what a tiara was.

"Maybe," I said, and I glanced down at my empty fingers and wrists resting on my thighs.

"Yeah, I know, you don't wear much jewelry. But we could find you something really nice for you, or big-time valuable." The thought of it made him happy; he beat his hand on the steering wheel to a song in his head.

"Well, we'll see what they have," I said, trying to sound excited.

"There it is—Greene Street," he said and made a left without using his blinker.

I couldn't believe that I had guessed the street, and it looked like we might be headed in the right direction. The number can't be right, I thought.

"You said 782?" he said.

"Yep, 782." I held my breath hoping it was the right number.

"It's on the left," he said, pulling to the side of the road facing the opposite direction of the other four cars that were there before us, even though the sun was just coming up. I could barely read the address, and I got it right.

A few pieces of furniture were lined up across the porch with three long folding tables in front of the house stacked with somebody else's things. Each had round white stickers marked neatly with $2.00, $.50, $1.75, and all other thought-out amounts that claimed the item's worth.

Behind the middle table sat a man and a woman each in a lawn chair with woven white and green webbing that was attached to metal frames that showed rust. The couple was old. She was thin with mostly silver hair with a patch of brown left from her younger self, and he wore a hat like the men did in the forties and fifties. I didn't doubt that the hat was made during the same time.

He was heavier and stayed in his chair, taking his hat off every few minutes, wiping the shine off his head with his handkerchief that he pulled out of his back pocket. She flitted from her squeaking chair and moved to different people, saying hello and asking if they had any questions. Her smile was wide and it filled her face with deeper wrinkles, making her somehow look younger. She was pretty.

"Good morning," she said to me and Vance.

"Good morning," I said, looking at her and imitating her smile. Vance moved on to another table scouting for gold.

"Did you have any questions on anything?"

"Not yet. You have some nice things," I said, not wanting her to walk off. I could feel her energy, the drive to move. I stood still, watching her fidget and smile and adjust things on the table. I wanted what she had; the power to move forward quickly without thinking.

"Are you moving?" I said. It was their home. No one had died. I was glad.

"Yes, we're moving to Alabama to live with our daughter and son. They both have their own families—so, each wants us for six months at a time, and then we move again."

I didn't want her to go.

"I went to Alabama when I was in eighth grade," I said.

"Not much different from here—is it?"

"No," I said.

"Keep looking. See if you like anything. I priced everything fairly," she said.

"I see that," I said. She found her way back to the middle table and made change for a lady who was buying a straw basket and porcelain painted elephant.

Vance was to the third table with nothing in his hands. We're going to have to buy something from this woman, I thought. I knew he was going to be ready to go as soon as he went through that table, and when he's ready, he's ready. I didn't want the day to turn ugly in front of those nice people.

I searched the table in front of me, picking up items to see what was underneath, hoping for something to buy. Purses lined most of the table, all in bright colors with wooden and cloth handles, all marked for $2.50 each. I wanted them all, but I knew Vance wouldn't have it. "What are you going to do with old lady purses?" he would say.

I chose the brightest one, so loud in orange and pink stripes that I could almost hear it singing to me. I picked up the purse, and underneath it was a necklace marked $3.00. It was costume with a gold chain and a round pendant on the end. It was plain compared to the purses. I wanted it. The lady walked toward me, and I paid her. Vance was watching—I hid the necklace from him and only showed it to her, tucking it inside the purse.

As he walked to the car, he said in a whisper, "Why did you buy that crazy-looking purse?"

"Why do you care?" I said and climbed in the car in a certain way that let him know that he couldn't stop me.

The lady had made me think about my trip to Alabama in eighth grade. As Vance drove us home, the memory grew stronger.

There was a set of double bridges that sit side by side in Alabama close to Mobile over a big river. It was raining heavy and Genesis was playing on Stephanie Blackwell's radio. Daniel was sitting in the seat in front of me next to this guy named Clay, and they were both pretending to play the drum part of the song. I watched as they beat on the seat in front of them. Daniel was the most animated, flailing his arms up and down hitting the seat with all the force a fourteen-year-old boy has. I felt sorry for Tammy Caruthers sitting in front of them. Clay was just following along, imitating the things that Daniel did. I looked up and saw the bridges ahead of us.

The tops were arched, and gables ran from top to bottom. As we rode over, I stared between the thick wires looking above the trees and power lines through the rain as the bus moved us toward Camp Moreland. I wanted to stop and stand on the edge of the bridge and absorb all of it in front of me. Even in the rain, I would have stood there.

I'd never been aware of so many beautiful things before me.

I was asleep on the way back and missed catching it for the last time.

Now, I stand above a pot of boiling potatoes. They're done, but I don't want to call Vance in here, yet.

I give CPR workshops every couple of months at the gym on Walnut Street next to Murphy's Eyeglass Shop. Dr. Kimberly suggested one day at work that I should get certified to teach it.

"You mean I am certifiable," I said, giving him a grin. He kept talking.

"It might be a good idea to show people something." He stood in the frame of the door that the patients come through. He's older, probably in his late sixties with thick white hair that curls in spirals all around his head. He tries to keep it short, but it turns wild the very next day after a haircut.

"I don't have that many things to show," I said. I placed my supplies on the counter, getting ready for the day. The doors were locked, and we were the first two people to arrive. We always are. I can't wait to get out of the house, and he breathes his job. From the age of eight, he knew what he was meant to do. I've been working for him for about two-and-a-half years now. I had worked for another doctor who only treated kids. It was too much, and I had to move on to Dr. Kimberly's. He only sees adults.

I take blood from all his patients. Nobody gets out of a doctor's office without having blood drawn.

He adjusted his bow tie—he wears one every day—well, every day that I see him, which is at work. It rests above his lab coat collar seeming to hold the jacket in place.

"I checked your appointments. You're going to be slammed," I said.

"Yep, if that's true, it will be the same for you, Tambri." He walked off in the direction of his office, looking back at me for a second.

I've come to dread the workshops. I've only taught for a short time, but there is always the same woman in each session. Not the exact same person, but always the same kind of woman; a young mother with her first child safe at home with the father. She is so afraid that the child is going to choke on a penny or pebble that the kid might stick in his mouth.

There she was this morning; I spotted her as I walked through the left side of the double-doors of the gym. This one was slender and cute with immaculate clothes, so neat. I could tell nothing bad had ever happened to her in her life.

She was part of a group of eight, five women and three men. Some were talking a little when I walked in, but mostly they were being quiet. Each one was nervous about learning such a serious thing, and afraid of looking stupid trying to learn something so important. I called the class together, and the young mother moved to the front with her shoes tightly laced, bouncing on her heels.

I used to be her.

"Mrs.—" she said right away.

"Just Tambri," I said and walked towards the locker where the instruction doll was.

"I am so glad I signed up for this class."

"Good," I said, stretching the doll on the waxed floor. If she only knew how weary I was from enthusiasm like hers. What good does it do her? Or me? I straightened myself and put my hands on my waist, daring anyone to speak. I smiled and looked around the class to make sure everyone was paying attention. It was then that I realized I knew one of the other women. She was in the very back of the class, and she seemed to be almost hiding from me.

"Georgette, is that you?" I said. Her husband had been a good friend of my first husband. I guess he still is. She inched forward a little and stood there in the class wearing wide pants that stopped at her knees. She wasn't wearing any makeup, and her sandy hair hung to her waist. She's always been religious; the kind of religious that doesn't believe in makeup or long pants for women. If anyone needs makeup—it's Georgette. And her round hips seemed to protrude through the heaviness of her culottes.

She made me think about when the four of us went to dinner a couple of times. The funny thing was that her husband Nicolas could care less about the church. I don't know if he'd ever gone to church in his life. He sat there with us drinking vodka and tonics like they were holy water. Georgette's mouth pursed more and more with each drink.

"You know you don't need that," she'd say.

"No, but I sure do want it," Nicolas would say and pour the drink he had down even faster. Georgette eventually would stop talking at all toward the end of the evening. Things always ended with Nicolas in the passenger seat of their car laughing and waving to us as she took off down the road. Like I said, we only went out with them a couple of times.

I haven't seen Georgette or her husband since things ended between me and Daniel. It was good to see her, and I had to hug her. Her body was limp, and I had the feeling that she wanted to pull away. I guessed that she felt strange about everything. It was just odd, though, because like I said, most women hug me with everything they have in their bodies.

"How's Nicolas?" I said.

"He's good."

"You still working at the Temp Agency?"

"Yep," she said. I couldn't figure her out. She's always been kind of strange, but not somebody that didn't want to talk.

"Tambri, if there's too many people in the class—I can come back another time," she said.

"No, it's fine. This is a good size group," I said. I get it, Georgette, is what I wanted to say. She wouldn't even look at me much. Ridiculous. I'm the one who's had it rough, why should she feel embarrassed? If embarrassed was even the right word for the way she was acting.

"Okay, let's get started," I said, and bent to the floor and lifted the head of the doll. Everyone formed a half-circle above me. One of the guys in a neatly tucked striped button-down shirt was taking notes already. What could he have possibly written down up to this point? I thought. Maybe he was writing down the conversation between me and Georgette.

"Everyone, this is Sally," I said.

"Hi, Sally," said the one with the tennis shoes. I'd almost forgotten about her.

"I have a question before we get started, if you don't mind?" she said, wanting to appear timid. I started thinking I should give her a little bit of a break. She was just trying to learn something that I was supposed to be there to teach.

"That's okay. What's your name?"

"Rebecca Waters."

"Rebecca is a pretty name," I said. I figured I'd make an effort to be friendly. "My first husband was a Waters."

I couldn't help but look over at Georgette since she knows all this. Her cheeks glowed; they were so red. "Tambri, I'll go first if you want me to," she said with the dumbest look on her face. What is wrong with her? I thought. She wanted to leave and barely spoke to me and then she volunteered to go first.

"Okay, Georgette," I said.

"Let me explain a few things, first. Make sure to use the antiseptic wipes on Sally before and after you resuscitate her. Okay?"

Everyone nodded or said yes.

"If not, you'll be kissing Sally along with everyone else in the group. And, I'm not sure if anyone wants that."

"Not me," said Georgette laughing. She just kept getting weirder.

"Sally can't breathe—so, your job is to do her breathing for her until help arrives," I said ignoring Georgette. She was beginning to annoy the hell out of me. I gave her this look to kind of tell her that she needed to calm down. She was looking back and forth between me and

Rebecca. Back and forth, almost like she was trying not to look back and forth, trying to show me something and not show me something.

And, then—I looked at Rebecca.

Rebecca is Daniel's second wife? I thought.

I looked at Georgette, and I knew it was true because she stopped looking at me and looked between the floor and Sally. Then I was the annoying one looking back and forth, except it was between Rebecca and Georgette.

Calm down, is what I kept thinking. I sat back on my heels, wiping the dolls mouth, staring at the alcohol as it clung to her rubber lips.

"You really want to make sure this area is clean," I said. I'm remarried; he's remarried. I knew that he had gotten married again about six months ago, and that's all there was. I had remarried first. There was no reason for him not to get married again. We both made our choices.

This is going to be fine, I thought. I focused on what my task was; it was good that I had something to do, something else to concentrate on.

"Georgette, come on over here. As I show you, I'll be teaching everyone else." I glanced at Rebecca again. I couldn't stop myself. She took this as a sign to ask her question that she didn't get to ask earlier.

"Do you have smaller ones to instruct on?" she said, smiling like a damn cat. I knew it—she has kids—this must be her second marriage, too. Georgette stopped walking in my direction.

"Come on over, Georgette. It's fine." I grinned at her trying to let her know that I had figured it out, but she was still unsure. Georgette moved forward, and Rebecca started talking again.

"It's just—"

"You want to make sure your kids are safe if they swallow something they shouldn't. Right?"

"Exactly," she said, bouncing on her heels again.

"Don't worry. I can show you everything with Sally. The timing is just a little different. We'll go through all that." Did I sound irritated? "Your kids will be fine under your watch," I said adjusting my tone.

"I don't have any, yet."

Out of the side of my eye, I could see Georgette's brown loafers stop moving. The muscles in her calves seemed to tighten.

"Any what?" I said tilting Sally's head.

"Kids. But we are trying," she said bouncing even faster.

I dropped Sally's head hard on the floor.

I looked at Georgette, and she had turned toward the gym door, almost like she was thinking of making a run for it. She twisted her body away, pretending to cough. She acted as if she was clearing whatever was lodged so deep in her throat.

Maybe it's penny or a pebble, I thought.

I turned my head away from the group, and toward the door that Georgette seemed mesmerized by. It was open, stuck on the rubber stopper outside. The light streamed in. Looking through, I could see Daniel's green truck. He fixed it up with his daddy's help. It was a wreck before that; today it looked brand new.

The starch explodes out of the potatoes, twirling in circles with the burning water. I put my hand in both pockets, touching the dolls with one hand, and the pretty old lady's necklace in the other. The necklace has been in my sweater ever since I bought it. The materials and shapes are so opposite from one another. I turn them over and over in my pockets while pieces of potatoes turn in the boiler.

"Is it almost ready?" Vance walks in the kitchen.

"Yeah, I just need to drain the water and add cream and mash them up. You know how I make potatoes." I lift the boiler and move it to the sink on the other side of the kitchen.

I open a couple of cabinets, looking for the colander.

"What else are we having?"

"What do you mean?" I really just want him to go back to the living room while I finish with everything.

"Besides mashed potatoes," he says.

I hadn't even thought about that. He said potatoes and that was what I was making him.

"We can make sandwiches," I say.

"I had a bad sandwich at lunch," he says.

"This one won't be bad."

I stick my hands back in my pockets without thinking as I walk back across the kitchen to check another cabinet.

I twist the dolls.

"What are you messing with in your pocket?"

I open another cabinet, pulling out the colander. He sees whatever I don't want him to see.

"Tambri?" he says, pushing it, wanting to know what I have in my pocket.

"Nothing, Vance," I say moving back to the sink, placing the colander on the opposite side of the sink from the potatoes.

I turn around, facing Vance, both my hands back in each pocket protecting the contents.

He walks over and forces his body against mine and pushes me against the sink. I feel the steam from the water on my shoulders as he forces me back without using his arms or hands, just the weight of his torso.

"What you got, Tambri?"

"Stop it," I say.

"Show me what you got in your pocket." He's maybe an inch from my face, bending me backwards more toward the sink. I feel the heat of the steam rising onto my neck.

"Let me go," I say, keeping my voice at an even level.

"Show me," he says. "Now."

I pull my dolls out of my right pocket and leave the other hand where it is.

I hold the dolls right up to his face.

He lets me loose and backs up staring at them. "What the hell are those? Some kind of voodoo dolls?" He moves farther back.

"Are you kidding me?" I say. I lean forward to see if I can make him move more. He does, and I almost want to laugh.

"You get rid of those things," he says.

I dangle one in front of him with blue pants and a white paper shirt. "This is you."

He bolts toward me. "Get rid of those damn things."

He grabs for me, and we start this chase in the small kitchen. I do laugh at this man who's scared of dolls, and it doesn't help his temperament at all. He starts lunging toward me.

"You know I'm going to eventually get you," he says breathing hard, sweat on his forehead.

"Yeah," I say, still running. I'm still laughing, and I'm not sure why. I can't seem to control it. Vance stops moving. And I stop, back at the side of the sink. We've both become quiet except for the sound of breathing. The dolls are suffocating in my closed damp hand.

He steps slowly towards me, knowing that I'm trapped.

I hold my hand above my head like I'm playing with a child.

He charges me. I turn to face the sink and drop the dolls into the hot water.

He watches them for just a second as they float on top of the water. "Why'd you do that?" He pulls back and walks out of the kitchen and into the living room, giving a low whistle.

"You are crazy, Tambri," he says loud enough for me to hear, and falls into his chair, turning the T.V. back on.

The reds and purples bleed from the dolls clothes, mixing, turning in the water. I turn the gold necklace in my pocket. The dolls float until the water soaks through, and they sink when the weight becomes too much.

Third Husband

It's loud as usual and The Allman Brothers are blaring over the speakers, but I can still hear the rattle of glasses and beer bottles slammed down on tops of tables and bars. Jesup, the bartender, keeps it cold. Temperatures rise when there's liquor involved.

I used to be a bouncer here for about a year or so to make a little extra money. Now it's just a place for me to come to, a place to go when I'm not on the road.

"Clay, look," Jesup says as he points toward this young girl probably just old enough to be in the bar. She's sitting with another girl who's got about twenty extra pounds on her.

Mark Jesup is the kind of guy that likes to lay it on thick when he's standing far enough away from the ladies. Always talking about how they're looking at him. He makes stories bigger than they are.

"I bet she'd go home with me, man."

"Yeah?" I was hoping he'd leave it alone. I'd rather talk about something else, but I know there's nothing I can do to stop him from running his mouth. Asshole.

"Yeah, can't you tell? She keeps eyeballing me from over there."

It's obvious that girl isn't interested in anybody in this place. She's holding her head down, doing most of the talking to her friend. She looks upset. It's got to be over a boyfriend. Something's happened. Her friend's trying to make her feel better.

I feel sorry for the girl. I feel sorry for both of them.

"You're crazy, man. That girl's upset about something." I'm trying to keep the vulture away from her. That's all the girl needs is some married bartender, grinning at her with false teeth.

"She isn't upset with me."

"Leave her alone, man," and I give him a look. He walks away cleaning the counter; he knows not to push it anymore. He knows how I handle things.

A couple of years back, there was a trucker who cut me off all the time. I don't drive like that; I try to help the other guys on the road with me. I tried to see if this guy was a jerk to everybody and he was kind of, but he really had it in for me. Sometimes that's the way it goes when you're the biggest guy in the room or on the road; somebody always wants to pick a fight.

This trucker's name was Thompson—I can't remember his first name—but one day I caught him saying shit on the CB to one of his buddies about me and my truck. He started again and weaved in and out in front of me. He always looks dirty, and he's the kind of guy that would blame it on truck driving, but that isn't so. There are plenty of places to stop and clean up. He's just too lazy to do it.

Finally, he pushed me over the edge, and I confronted him at Jack and Jill's rest stop on 92 in Vidalia. I was hauling onions to South Carolina. He said some things. When I got closer to him, he'd back up and say, "I don't want to fight."

Then he'd make another remark while I was walking away.

I ended up walking over to him, and I got right in his face. "Is there something else you want to say to me? You better do it while I'm standing here, because if I hear you say one more thing while I'm walking back to my truck, I'm going to turn back around and punch you right in your ugly nose."

"No, why you trying to start something?" he said, all innocent like.

"I'm not the one running my mouth. Say one more thing and I'll finish it for you."

"I don't have a gripe with you," he said. His red hat sat sideways on his head. He's way too old to have it cocked that way.

I turned around, and he said something under his breath. I couldn't make it out, but I knew it was smartass.

I had my fist up before I turned back around. I connected without even trying.

He took me to court, and I spent three weeks in jail. Two months on probation and I almost lost my CDL license. I broke his cheekbone in two places.

To say I'm direct when it comes to that kind of thing is kind of funny. I wish I was more that way when it came to women. Not the hitting, of course, just the getting things out and taking care of it.

I drink the last swallow from my Bud Lite. I've been trying to lose a few pounds. Sitting in a truck all day doesn't do much for your waistline. Not that I'm fat. I guess most people describe me as husky. Six foot two, two hundred and fifty pounds, yeah, I guess most people call that husky. At least that's what they call me to my face.

Jesup brings me another beer, and I turn toward the door to watch people coming in. It's Saturday evening, and I can see that the sunlight is almost gone as people pull open the door and it shuts behind them. Picking up in here. It makes me feel better to be around people. You know how some people like to stay at home and not go out. I like to get out and just see people. Truck driving isn't the best choice for my kind of personality, I guess, but I like it, too.

There's a woman coming through the door. The light is right behind her and I can't quite make her out, but the look of her is familiar to me. There's a guy coming in behind her. I watch and wait for the door to slam back, to see if I can make her out. It shuts and I have to give it a second for my eyes to adjust from the last light outside to the dark inside here. I wait as she comes into focus.

It's Tambri.

Three years since I've seen her. Me and her first husband were always good friends. All of us have known each other since high school. I'd go over to their house on weekends, when I was in town, and we'd grill out. Then their little boy passed away. They got divorced because of it.

I've missed her.

I know who that is with her. It's that son-of-a-bitch of a second husband of hers. I could not believe it when I heard they got married. The idea of it worries me.

I wait for her to see me, making sure my shirt is tucked into the back of my pants. She is lovely. I heard some English guy use that word in a movie and it fits Tambri. Lovely.

She lifts her head of shiny brown hair and twists the ends with her fingers. She's always done that, especially when she's feeling out of place.

I really knew Tambri before Daniel did. I saw her before I met her in high school. She was probably eleven at the time. She used to come over to her grandma's house during the summers once in a while and spend the night. Her grandma lived next door to my house.

I'd see her jumping on the trampoline that her grandmother had bought for her. I'd always try to get up the nerve to walk over to the fence and say something, but all I could manage was a wave, and that was always when she was jumping. I knew she could only wave and wasn't able to say much back.

Then in eighth grade she showed up in my first session biology class. There were only eight people in the class. Me and Tambri and this one guy that everybody thought might be gay—later on turned out he was. This girl named Susan that came from Mattie Pye Elementary, just like me, and a few other kids I don't really remember now. Not that it was a small school. It was the higher level class and only a few qualified to be in it after grammar school. Science was my best subject, and Tambri always did well in everything.

I talked to her more in junior high and high school. We were usually in the same science class up until about the eleventh grade. Then they brought in more teachers for science, and I ended up separate from her.

She was always sweet to me. I guess she was that way toward everybody. I never had a chance with her back then, and I ended up going to prom with Michelle Tisdale. She was pretty enough and nice enough, but she wasn't Tambri.

Tambri went with Daniel. He was a nice guy, and we played football together. They married right out of high school. It was sad when it ended for them. Even though I've always thought about her more than I should, I really wanted them to make it. Do the old age thing together.

Me and Michelle thought about getting married. But I don't know, it just never felt right to me. I loved her and everything; I just couldn't see having kids with her. She was kind of spoiled, which isn't so bad. Her daddy had a little money from his rental properties, and she had four older brothers, so, of course, she was his favorite.

I knew she'd end up treating our kids the way her daddy treated her. It's all she knew; why would she change when we had kids? I'm out on the road most of the time hauling watermelons or cotton or shoes or something. Those kids would be out-of-control by the time I got back.

Hell, I don't know, maybe I didn't love her.

My dad had a stroke at the end of my senior year. He was only forty-nine at the time. He's a big guy like me. He survived it, but I had to help out and that's when I started truck driving. I worked for Randall Jones for about five years, moved around for a while from company to company.

I drive for myself now, whatever I can get to haul, and I like being on my own anyway. Some of the owners try to force you to drive longer than you're supposed to, or load the truck heavier than you're supposed to.

Man, I'm just not into taking those kinds of chances. It'll be my butt that's burned, and in the second place, it's not right to begin with. You'd be surprised how many trucks are driven by guys that are more than tired and jacked up on whatever they could get their hands on.

I'm wishing Tambri would walk over. I keep watching, hoping she can feel me looking at her. Vance has got his arm around her, trying to keep her beside him. She's skinny. That bothers me. I'm sure Mr. Wonderful isn't helping matters any. He's a hard worker and everything, fixing copiers, but I've always heard things about the way he treats women. You can't keep that kind of stuff quiet.

I've taken jobs that kept me on the road for long periods of time so that I wouldn't accidentally bump into Tambri in town somewhere. I couldn't stand to see her so sad. I had to run into her eventually, and there she is walking towards me. And now I'm wondering as I see her beautiful face: Why did I hide?

I'm waving and grinning at her, and she walks into my arms and hugs me. It's the warmest hug, and I know that her eyes are closed, even though I can't see them. My throat sticks as I try to say her name. I can feel what she's been through in the tininess of her waist, and how her breath comes ragged onto my neck.

Vance stopped at two other tables, talking to his asshole friends. Saying how good his wife looks; letting them stare at her. I wouldn't put up with it, and I wouldn't treat her like that, but she's not my wife.

"It's good to see you, Tambri."

"You, too, Clayton," she says smiling big at me. She's one of the few people besides my mother who still calls me that. She smoothes down the sides of her dress with her hands. The dress is black and it fits close, stopping right above her knees. The black overwhelms her body.

"You look wonderful, Tambri," I say, kind of choking again.

She smiles because she knows I'm not trying to get anything from her.

"You always make me feel good, Clay." It feels like no time has gone by. We have that kind of friendship; it makes me wish I'd gone to see her before now instead of running into her at a bar.

Vance is headed over. He couldn't let her stand here next to me for too long.

"Hey, big boy." Apparently, he can't remember my name.

"Hey, man," I say.

"You over here trying to steal my girl?"

"No, she walked over to see me. I guess she wanted to see a friendly face."

He lets that one go.

"You still hauling for Jacob and Sons?"

"No. Out on my own now," I say.

He's halfway listening. He's really trying to figure out how to get Tambri away from me and back to his table. He can't tell her she has to come back to his table, although I can see that he sure wants to. He knows she'd probably say no, and then it would start something with me, and that is the last thing he wants.

"Tambri, let's sit over here, honey," Vance says. That's right—sweeten it with the honey.

"No, I want to talk to Clay for a while."

"You don't mind a couple of old friends talking, do you?" I say. This is beginning to be a little fun.

"Of course not, she can stand here all night long if she wants to."

He backs up and sits with a couple of guys I've seen here before. Safety in numbers. Plus, he doesn't want to look like a jackass sitting by himself, while his wife talks to an old friend that knows her better than he ever will.

He orders a beer and checks out the waitress's ass. He knows me and Tambri are watching him. That's part of the game for him, to show her how far he will go, which makes me sick to think about. Tambri deserves better.

"Are you doing okay, Clay?" She turns and sits on the stool next to me. Vance keeps his eye on us as he drinks and seethes. He's moving around in his chair like he can barely take the feel of the cushion under his butt.

He can stare all he wants. She's made her choice and her choice right now is me. It would be so easy to walk over and push his face into the table, but Tambri wouldn't want that. I'll rein it in just for her. Besides, I'm the one sitting elbow to elbow with her, close enough to smell her skin. This is so much better than punching that asshole in the face.

"Yeah, happy to see you," I say, turning to look at Tambri directly.

"Me, too."

"Yeah."

I glance down, out of embarrassment, I guess. She left her shoes on the floor when she sat down. One black shoe is turned on its side while the other stands alone. Her feet exposed. I look at her red toenails, and she sees me.

"Vickie did my toes for me."

"Oh," I say lifting my head back up. "Is she still working at the hair salon?"

"Yeah, she's at the same place."

She rests her feet on the bottom rung of the stool. She looks so clean, and I keep thinking that not any part of her should touch the nasty floor. She shouldn't be in here at all, around all this dirtiness.

She's so pale now; she used to always be tan. Always riding her horses. She tried to teach me how to ride when we were both about sixteen.

You could tell she knew what she was doing on that horse. Tambri sat with her back so straight. She laughed the whole time we were riding, and I'm pretty sure it was because of me. I have no coordination when it comes to that kind of thing. I remember bouncing and bouncing on that poor horse—its name was Rosie. Poor Rosie. I felt bad that she carried all my weight, and I didn't know what the hell I was doing, sitting on top of that horse bouncing all the way. Tambri laughing behind me.

"I know I look funny on this thing."

"No, you don't. You look manly."

"That's a good way to put it." I liked that she had called me manly. When you're sixteen, being called a man makes you feel good. Makes you feel protective of the pretty girl who said it.

We both sit quiet at the bar, each of us thinking about things.

She touches my hand just for a second. "You remind me of everything good."

"Like me riding a horse?" I smile at her.

"Yep," she says laughing low.

"It was funny."

"You never give yourself enough credit, Clay." She says my name real soft. I cough to cover the well that's opened up inside me. My face feels hot.

She's still trying to make me feel good. I want to reach over, and hold her for a long time, and not say anything.

He watches us. So easy to read the way he leers at all the women, bringing his eyes back to her once in a while; demanding that she come back in his silent, useless way.

"I'm worried that you may be asking for it, tonight," I say.

"It doesn't matter what I do. If it's not tonight, it'll be tomorrow night," she says, looking away from me, moving the tips of her fingers along the bar's surface. My stomach churns to hear her confirm what I already knew, still I don't move from where I'm sitting.

She leans in closer to me. Not looking me in the eye, looking down at the dark wood of the bar.

"You should be with me, just for a while." I whisper the words, and I've never said anything like that to her.

She puts her hand around my upper arm and lays her cheek against my shoulder. She exhales and her warm breath moves down my arm and burns my skin. I sit stone still as I feel her give in.

"Wally, how about a beer?" she says to Jesup as she pulls away.

"It's Jesup," he says smiling at her.

"Hey, Jesup. Wally is what I call bartenders."

"Yeah, why's that?"

"I don't know. It's just something silly to say. The guy always ends up telling you his name, and then you never have to call him bartender."

She's messing with Jesup. He doesn't really know how to take it. He decides to change the subject.

"You a friend of Clay's?"

"Looks like it, Jesup."

The Movement
of Feral Cats

"Hand me the hammer," Clay says. I sit on top of the house next to him while he kneels replacing shingles on the roof. I pick up the hammer and turn it in my palm; they don't make them as strong as this anymore. Clay's had it since he was seven. He takes it, using the claw to pull old nails out. He sticks the nails into his front jean pocket.

"Don't forget you put those in there," I say. "I don't want to hear you yelling later because you've stuck them into your thigh." I smile at him, shielding my eyes from the brightness. The sun bounces into his face, and he picks up the white towel that he's brought with him and wipes his neck and hands.

"Do you want me to get you a hat? Your old grey one's in the living room closet," I say.

"No, it just makes me hotter." He pulls the old shingles off like paper and tosses them out to the sky. They stick together as they fall fast and collide with the ground.

I bend my legs, resting my head sideways on top of my knees toward Clay, winding my arms around my calves.

"You make me nervous being up here," he says, nails hanging from his mouth, "Especially with shorts and sandals on."

"I'm fine, Clay, do you know how tall a horse is when you ride one? Roxie is sixteen hands high."

"Is Roxie as high as a one-story house?"

"I promise I'll sit right here and not even move a toe." I squeeze my legs tighter with my arms.

"You better sit still, woman." He threatens me with a crooked smile of teeth and nails.

I look out and see the horses moving into the barn, almost as if they hear the conversation and want no part of it. They move at a leisurely pace with Roxie leading, Chester and Benji following. The heat is probably too much for them right now. They'll head back out in a couple of hours.

Sammy named Benji. My first husband, Daniel, and I had gone to pick the horse out when Sammy was two-and-a-half. I wanted him to grow up riding. We had just rented the dog movie *Benji* a couple of days before. Sammy watched it four times.

"Benji is a dog name," Daniel said looking down at our son as I held him.

Sammy leaned forward, and patted the horse on its white nose. "I love Benji," he said.

"Son, what about Thunder or Lightning?" Daniel was beginning to beg. "Don't you want your horse to have a tough name?"

I rocked back and forth in slow motion with Sammy in my arms, smiling at Daniel's weak attempts. I kissed Sammy on the head and laughed into his hair.

"Of course you think this is funny. You named the other two before we were even here, before Sammy was even born. Roxie sounds like an eighty-year-old stripper and Chester is a holier-than-thou English guy with a damn pipe in his mouth."

"Daniel, you told him he could name it whatever he wanted."

"That was before you let him watch that movie!"

He grumbled while he loaded Benji into the trailer.

It's strange what men want control of.

"Those are really short," I say to Clay, pointing at the nails as he hammers them in.

He stops and looks at me. "They only have to be long enough to go through the shingle and then a little ways through the roof." He continues hammering.

I look around, high above everything. I see the cats inching their way out of the protection of the trees. "Clay, your feral cats are coming out of the woods."

He stands straight, turns around, and watches. I can see he wants them to go to the food he has put out. They only live a few years, and he wants to change that for the small group heading toward our house. They won't come near it if we're outside and on the ground. This is the first really good look I've ever gotten of them.

All five of them are striped different shades: black, orange, white, grey, tan. They all have narrow eyes. The orange and white one, towards the back, only has one eye. They move with caution and flinch at the smallest leaf. Their fur is wild and looks sticky compared to regular cats. I guess survival is more important than grooming. I can feel Clay holding his breath beside me as they move closer to the house and the food. You can't pet them or anything. Clay gives to them and gets nothing back.

"This is the closest they've ever been to the food," Clay says in a whisper.

There is noise from the barn, and Benji tromps outside toward them, and they scatter back to their hiding places.

"Damn it," Clay says. He kneels and shakes his head as he continues to nail shingles.

"They'll come back," I say.

"I guess. They don't look good from here."

"How are they supposed to look?" I try to find them in the woods, where they've disappeared. Maybe I see a pair of eyes looking back?

"I'm not sure, but I thought they seemed skinny."

"Don't they learn how to take care of themselves?"

"I just wanted to help them out a little."

"I know," I say.

I knew Clay from before anything bad had happened to me. No child had been born or died. No divorce from the man that I should have been married to all my life. He was good friends with Daniel. Maybe that's why I picked him next.

Sometimes, he'll say things the way that Daniel did before we divorced. "We are good to go," or "nice one," Clay will say holding the word "one" for a couple of seconds. It could be a smart remark, like when I accidentally put a fresh container of chocolate ice cream in the refrigerator.

He opened the door two hours later and found it. He walked it to the side door of the house and outside where I was cleaning out my car. He made sure that I gave him my full attention and saw the thawed carton before he said a word.

"Nice one," he said. He laughed deep, and the lines around his eyes curled upward.

"Well, damn," I said, and laughed with him. He tossed it in the plastic bag I was using for trash and helped me finish my car. He turned on the radio, and we both sang *Take it to the Limit* as we sprayed the windows with cleaner and used the rest of the roll of paper towels.

"I bet those cats are miles away if they can hear our singing," Clay said. I sang louder in the car, and Clay made a howling noise.

It wasn't the end of the world or anything like that with Clay. He doesn't let those kinds of things bother him.

Now, it's not a good thing to make Clay angry; not that he gets angry often. He's the kind that it takes a lot—but when he's pushed, he'll push back and hard.

When we first got married, Vance, my second husband, came by drunk as I've ever seen him. Me and Clay were inside the house. I was reading a magazine, and Clay was changing out the filter for the air conditioner. I didn't even hear a car pull up. And then this beating started at the door. I knew who it was.

I stood and looked down the hallway at Clay. He was pulling the old air filter out. His jaw tightened, but he refused to look at me. He'd heard it, too. His plan was to ignore it until the noise stopped, and Vance went away. I sat down again and pretended to read. I remember staring at a picture of pecan-encrusted tilapia with green beans. Looking at it made me nauseous.

The knocking went on. Two loud beats and then nothing, like Vance was standing there waiting for a response. Then three beats, louder. Demanding that someone open the door. He wasn't going anywhere.

I decided I'd better go to the door first and try to make him leave. He didn't want Clay coming to the door. I thought he must be drunk to show up here with Clay in the house.

Two more loud beats sounded. The noise went through me as I crossed the kitchen.

I unlocked the door and eased it open. The screen door was still locked, and I saw where he'd dented the metal frame with his fist.

There he stood with no shirt on and behind him stood his buddy, Frankie Watson. As bad as Vance is, Frank is worse. Somebody said he pulled a knife on a guy once. Who knows if all of it is true. Some of it's got to be true. I do know that he sent this teenage kid to the hospital. I talked to Linda Truetlen, the boy's mother, a couple of weeks afterwards and she said, "Tim was doing much better, but when it first happened they wondered if he would make it." People don't make up that many stories unless some truth got them started.

Frank was the reason that Vance knocked on the door with such hatred and bravery. It was his buddy Frank.

I crossed my arms in front of me and peered through the screen at the two drunk men that stood on the other side.

"What do you want, Vance?" I said.

"He wants your husband to come outside," Frankie said laughing. I ignored him and searched for Vance's truck or some kind of vehicle.

"How'd you get here, Vance?" I said, saying Vance's name loud so Frankie wouldn't get confused and try to answer for him.

"Cheryl Ramsey dropped us off down the road," Vance said.

"Yeah, we told her we wanted to sneak up on you and your husband," Frankie said.

"So, you're telling me that you assholes don't have a way home?" I said.

Neither one of them said anything. They looked at each other, and they laughed and snorted and slapped their legs.

"Man, I didn't even think about that," Frankie said.

"Me neither, man," Vance said. "Tambri, can you give us a ride home?"

Frank loved that. I thought he might throw up he was laughing so hard.

"It's the middle of the day. How'd you two get wasted so early?" It was Clay talking then. He'd walked up behind me without me knowing. I could feel his breath on the top of my head. I froze like one of his cats.

Frankie stood up straight. "None of your business," he said as he moved back little by little. He looked like he was getting ready to run. But where would he go? He was way too messed up to find his way through the woods.

Vance was still too full of Wild Turkey to realize the danger in front of him.

"I came to see you, Clay," he said. He pointed his finger at Clay and his hand wavered with the weight of liquor.

"Yeah," Frankie said, standing several feet behind Vance and moving farther back as he spoke.

Clay pushed past me and hit the door so hard with his open palm that it swung out making the hair on Vance's head move with the wind. Vance backed up.

Clay stood over him waiting for him to do anything. Vance stood still. There was finally fear in his face. He was realizing how big Clay was, how much he had pushed Clay by coming to his house and bothering his wife. He knows Clay loves me and will defend me, even though I don't love Clay. Well, not the way a husband should be loved.

I felt bad for Vance. He hadn't thought this thing through.

"Clay, this was a bad idea," Vance said, staring at Clay's chin.

"Yep," Clay said, moving towards him.

Vance turned and ran. The three of us, Clay, Frankie, and me watched him as he ran out toward the horse corral. I walked out of the house and me and Clay both walked past Frankie and headed toward where Vance was.

"Ah, man," Frankie said in a low voice as I stepped beside him. He was upset, I guess, because it didn't look like there was going to be a fight that day.

Vance stood in the corral, and the horses moved around him. Vance turned in a circle facing out, looking at each horse. He tripped over nothing, it looked like, and then he ended up on the ground sitting on his butt.

"Damned dandelions," he said, pulling at the weeds around him. He let go of the grass and let himself fall back first into the dirt. Benji touched Vance's face with his nose.

"Hey, Benji," he said, looking into the horse's nostrils. Vance wasn't able to get up by himself. Maybe Benji was trying to help.

We stood at the fence. I looked through the two upper slats at Vance on the ground and Clay looked over at him.

"Are you okay?" Clay said.

"Yeah, the world's spinning around me. I'm going to be sick before this day is over."

Clay put his hand on the upper slat of the fence getting ready to climb through. And then, Frankie was there.

He had a pointed end of a bottle opener sticking out of his hand and he caught the upper part of Clay's arm. He pushed the metal into Clay's skin and left it there to hang in the muscle.

Clay made a painful noise that I won't forget. The blood running from his arm scared me. I went after Frankie.

I stopped in front of him determining what to do.

"I don't want to hurt no woman, but I will if you keep coming towards me, Tambri," he said.

His words pushed me forward and all I could think was, I want to hurt him. I lunged at him with my hands balled into the tightest fists I could make, and I hit him in his face with the front and sides of my closed hands. We stood together in a kind of violent hug. I felt him hitting me in the back. I'd been hit before. This time with every one of his punches, I'd hit him in his nose, his mouth, his forehead. I was looking up into his face as I attacked him, and I could see blood forming in the left opening of his nose, and I hit that side as hard as I could and the blood poured out and onto my hand. It seemed like this went on for the longest time, but it had to be just a few seconds. Everything seemed to just about stop. It was easy to hit him—like he had targets painted on his face.

Clay's hands wrapped around my waist, pulling me gently away from Frankie. I remember my feet swinging above the ground as he moved me away.

He brought Frankie down with one punch to his neck. Frankie threw his hands to his throat covering where Clay had made contact. He was trying to say stop, but Clay had punched his voice right out of him. All that came out was a pathetic sound of choking breath. He lay on the ground like he was done. Clay pulled him back up by the shoulder seams of his shirt. Blood ran from Clay's arm. The pain seemed to provoke him more. It was with that arm that he punched and lifted Frankie for a second time before Frankie was able to fall to the safe earth. Clay would have gone on more, but he was worried about me, and I'd marked Frankie pretty good. It's easy to beat up a drunk son-of-a-bitch when he's left his weapon in someone else's arm.

Everybody ended up going to the emergency room together; Clay with his arm, me with my back, and Frankie with his ugly face.

Frankie took Clay to court for it and said that he was protecting Vance. He had pictures and everything. Clay won—Frankie had pulled the bottle opener on him first. Nothing was mentioned about me.

I look over now at the scar on Clay's arm. He ended up having seven stitches. Nothing compared to Frankie.

I reach over and trace the scar on Clay's arm. Its shape reminds me of a dragon. But maybe I'm trying to make it seem like something tough. Maybe it just looks like a scar made by an idiot with a bottle opener. It does look like a snake. Or, maybe, a worm? He stops working and looks at me.

"Are you thinking about that, again," he says. He's laughing at me a little.

"What's funny about that is—I always thought you needed protecting. But you throw a pretty good punch."

"I learned from you."

"I've done worse things to myself driving my truck than this place on my arm, Tambri."

"Like bobtailing," I say. I've rode with him a couple of times in his truck when he wasn't hauling anything. Bumpiest, scariest ride I've ever taken. Well, besides being married to Vance.

"Yep, like bobtailing. Also, avoiding the lounge lizards at the truck stops." He laughs as he moves over to the other side of the triangle of the roof.

"I kind of feel sorry for those women, Clay."

"Yeah me, too. I tried to give one a ride one time and money to help her out…"

"And she tried to give you a ride?"

"Let's just say I bounced her right out of my truck at the next stop. I didn't want any part of that."

"Good for you," I say, trying to lean back more on the roof.

"I wish I had a palette up here," I say. "I'd lie all the way out on it."

He tosses me his sweaty towel, and I put it under my head.

"I remember in kindergarten that we had to lie on palettes after lunch and take a nap. Did you ever do that?"

"I think every kid has done that, Tambri." He's behind me now, and I hear his hammering and his voice in between.

"I was in Mrs. Simpson's class. She wasn't a very nice first teacher. I remember her being hateful to all the kids. She'd only be mean when they were no other adults in the room."

I try to put my legs flat out on the roof and pull them back in a hurry. The roof is hot now.

"I told you," Clay says as he stands above and behind me. "Do you want me to help you down off of here?"

"No," I say. "That was the year I had chicken pox."

"Yeah?" he says. He's barely listening. I guess he's trying to finish before the day's gone.

"The doctor thought I'd brought small pox back." I can feel that he's farther away from me at the outer corner of the roof. As far away as he can get from me at this point.

The hammering continues. I strain to see the cats moving out of the woods into the grey of the evening. I watch as they slink closer to Clay's bowls.

"Clay, the cats are here, again," I say in a whisper. I hear him slide more shingles off and to the ground on his side of the house. "Clay."

"It's okay, Tambri. I don't have to see them. I need to finish this."

Riding the Mythomania

"Take that plastic hat off," I tell her as she leans in to kiss me right on the mouth, right in public, right at the potato chip plant where she works. She yanks it off her head and squishes it in my face and lets it fall in my lap. She walks around the front of the car so I can watch her. She's got wide hips, and she likes to move them. She doesn't care that her ass is big. I look in my mirror to wipe her purple lipstick off my mouth; it sticks to the back of my hand.

"Thanks for picking me up," she says, climbing in the car. She slams the door, like she wants to break it at the hinges. Sometimes she tries to break me at the hinges.

She smoothes her hair with her fingers; it's wild from the hat. "How many days?" she says.

"I don't know." I run my hand up her leg, across her white pants.

"Yeah, you do. How many days until you get married, Kyle?"

"Twenty, twenty-one. Something like that."

"It's nineteen. We better make the most of it since we won't be seeing each other anymore." She laughs deep. "Take me home, baby."

I pull out fast and head to Doris' house. She lives three miles from the plant; I've clocked it. How fast can I get her home? Five-and-a-half minutes if I take Swanson Road.

"You smell like Ruffles," I say. I glance over, and she's pulling the visor down, checking her makeup in the mirror.

"Wonder how that happened?" she says, still looking in the mirror, turning her head from side to side to see herself from all angles.

Tambri doesn't wear makeup, not that I can tell anyway. Not the way Doris wears it.

"Shit, Kyle. There's a cop behind you," Doris says.

"Don't worry about it," I say in my soothing voice.

I've been stopped three times before, doing at least fifteen miles over the speed limit. Once on Parker Street, one time before on this road (Doris wasn't with me that time), and one time on I-75 right below Tifton, on my way to Florida, I was stopped by a state trooper. The last one I was a little concerned about. Phil Jordan, one of my drinking buddies, told me they could be hardnosed.

"Man, they will stick you to the wall if they stop you for speeding," he said. That was the last time I went out drinking with him. Apparently, he doesn't know his foot from his ear.

They didn't even give me a warning. I was inviting the guy over for dinner before it was all over. I've got caught, but no one's ever burned me.

"Is it anybody you know?" Doris says. She twists her neck to glance over the back seat, squinting her eyes to make him out.

"Not that I can tell," I say. It's a county car, and I do know a few of the deputies, but not this one. "Hand me my insurance card out of the glove box." I look back, and he's still sitting in his car. Good. I ease out of my car, license and insurance card in my left hand.

You always need to get out of the car before the cop comes to your door to get you. I walk to the back of my car, making sure not to block my tag that he's running right now.

Nothing there, Buddy, look all you want, you'll see nothing but clean. He's taking his time getting out of his car. Big guy, probably six-two, maybe in his early thirties like me, I can work with that; we already have something in common.

"How are you doing?" I say.

"License and insurance card, please."

"Right here, Officer. I'm sorry about the shape of the insurance card—my Lab got a hold of it."

"That's all right, Mr. Thomas, I can still see everything. Would you happen to know how fast you were going?"

"No, I can't say that I was paying as much attention as I should."

"It's somewhat important to pay attention when you're driving. Don't you think, Mr. Thomas?" He holds on to his ticket book. He hasn't decided what he was going to do with me yet.

"You are absolutely right about that. The fact is I just got engaged, and I guess I was concentrating on that." I give him this kid grin, like I'm unsure of the whole marriage thing.

"Is that her in the car?"

I look back at Doris whose smiling toward us with her neck still twisted. She'd enjoy this if she could hear it.

"Yep, that's her. She'll be Mrs. Doris Thomas." I laugh out loud at the thought of that. "It makes me a little nervous to think about."

"I've been married for seven years. Best thing that ever happened to me."

"That's good to hear. I know I've made the right decision, and that woman sitting in my car is the best thing that ever happened to me." I throw a wave to Doris, and she waves back.

"Well, I can't very well put a damper on your engagement, can I?"

"I sure would appreciate it if you didn't."

"Slow it down, then. You don't want anything to happen to your fiancé."

"No, sir."

"She like dogs, too?"

"Sir?"

"Does she get along with your Lab?"

"Yeah, she loves Jack."

"Good luck," he says walking back to his car, closing up his ticket book.

I get back in the car and tell Doris the story. She laughs so much, she's howling when she hears it. She starts coughing and finally has to stop.

Tambri laughs, but not like Doris. When Tambri does laugh, it doesn't cover her face, just the corners of her mouth and never her eyes. Doris laughs and the car shakes, and you can tell she's laughing just by looking at her, even if you couldn't hear—you could tell.

Me and Tambri were sitting out in her backyard the other night. Well, it's more like a pasture where she keeps her horses. The summer bugs were in full noise mode, and all you could hear was the sound they were making. Once in a while, one of her horses in the stalls would move around and make a noise. Other than that, it was quiet. We didn't talk for the longest time, and I reached over and took her hand; it was warm and small in my scratched up hand, and I felt calm when it was in mine.

"I'm happy," I said.

She smiled and kept looking straight ahead, her face sunburned from the first hot day of the year. It sneaks up on you like that sometimes. You think you're okay, and it's still spring, but then you're burned like a used up pack of matches. Her lips were swollen from the sun, and I had the urge to grab her like I do Doris. I held her hand tighter and turned from looking at her.

"How was work today?" I said.

"Fine, nothing unusual," she said.

I placed her hand back on the arm of her wooden chair, and I looked straight ahead, copying her.

"We didn't really have a spring, did we?" she said.

"I was just thinking that."

"I remember when the birds came out for the first time. It was so odd, all the noise that I heard. I walked out here, and they were everywhere, most of them finches, flying from tree to tree to Mr. Connelly's fence. I looked down, and they threw moving shadows on the ground. There was just a little warmth that day, and it was all they were waiting for."

I looked over, and it was like she could see it right in front of her. Memories sometimes seemed stronger to her than what was going on that moment.

She looked at me with a slight curl to the corner of her bruised lips. "It was almost like they were playing games, putting on a show to see who could make the most shade with their little bodies."

"Yeah?" I said. I couldn't see what she was seeing.

Lightning interrupted her; it was miles off, probably in Jefferson or Tateville.

"Hey," I said, "we should go fly a kite with a key on it."

She laughed, and it almost reached her eyes.

"No thanks, I think electricity has been invented for some time now." We watched the lightning for a while, but all she saw were the birds.

I shift the car into fourth and drive past Doris' road.

"Where are we going?"

"I thought we'd ride some. Where do you want to go, Cinderella?"

"Beats me, Prince."

We pass a cotton field on the right. It's the second pull from the cotton and the tops are dirty white. It's never as bright and clean as people think.

"Man, you fixed it with that cop," Doris says. She messes with the radio trying 95.6 and 99.4, then switches it to the

CD. She forgot she borrowed my Jamison CD without asking. There's nothing in there, and she turns it off.

"I guess so," I say.

When I was a teenager, I used to go get a job at the fair when it came into town. Man, it smelled so good, fried sausages, French fries, everything fried. I never did get to eat any of it. I usually ran late, and I couldn't eat while I was working, and everything was closed by the time we locked things up. Once in a while, the wind would shift, and the smell from the cows and pigs would drift over, then I didn't care about getting anything to eat anyway.

I worked the week of the fair for three or four years. I think my first fair was when I was about fifteen. There was always so much sound from the rides, and people talking and laughing, and the guy on the Discotheque screaming over the microphone, "Do you want to go faster!" to all the riders flying around over and over in the same circle. Yes, man, everybody wants to go faster.

I'd usually work at one of the games. Maybe, the crazy clowns with the balloons on top of their heads that people had to bust by shooting water in the clown's mouth, or, one year, I worked at the gold fish game.

We ran out of goldfish one time, and somebody went to K-mart and bought orchids for people to pitch for. They were pretty, but they really didn't draw people in that much, not the guys anyway. They wanted to win their girlfriends a huge stuffed animal, so their women would think of their men every time they looked at the big monkey or alligator.

This little girl came by with her mom and was looking at the orchids. You know how little girls are, they like everything with princesses and flowers. Her mom saw her looking.

"How much is it to play?" her mom said.

"Fifty cents, you get one throw per quarter," I said. It was a hard game; the goal was to land the quarter on this big table that had these bull's eyes all over it. It had to be dead center of one of the bull's eyes, and it was a small center, and we waxed the surface to make it even more slippery. When things got really busy those quarters would fly. Some people would end up spending ten dollars on something that was only worth about a buck-and-a-half.

The mother was pretty, and her face was flushed like she'd just scrubbed it with soap. Both of them had shiny blonde hair; they looked like something on T.V. Where was her husband? She had a ring on; he should be here with them, I remember thinking. The mother handed me a dollar, and I gave her four quarters. In all of twenty seconds, all four quarters were either sitting outside of a painted circle or in the dirt.

"Well, Mommy tried," she said. Her little girl shook her head. I could tell she was sad and really wanted one, even though she hadn't said a word.

They started to walk off and the girl looked around to see the orchids one more time. I picked one up and walked towards her. She moved closer to her mom and turned around. She wanted to be away from me more than to have the pretty flower.

"Hey," I said to the mom. "She can have this if she wants it."

"That's okay," her mom said. "I wouldn't want to get you in trouble with your boss." She pulled her daughter closer to her, gave the weakest smile, turned around and walked away from me. "I didn't win it," she was saying to her daughter. I looked for them to show up at the fair every year after that.

If you want to make Doris happy, tell her you're taking her to Savannah for the weekend.

"Doris, let's go out of town this weekend. How about Savannah?"

"Really? I haven't been there in such a long time. I think I was about twenty-two the last time I went there. We can go to Tybee Island, get a nice hotel to stay in, eat seafood and drink on River Street. "

"Okay, if you want to do all that, we can." That Doris knows how to live.

"I remember what was going on the last time I went. It was St. Patrick's Day, and I went there with a bunch of my friends; there was probably eight girls staying in the same room. Two to a bed, some of us on the floor. You know how it is when you're that young, and you don't care about sleeping on the floor with your friends."

"I like the sound of that," I say.

"Shut up. We would go out and flirt with the guys and get wasted on Hurricanes. This one lady had a big poodle that she had dyed green. That dog looked pitiful, the dumb animal. I wonder if it just sat there and took it while the woman was pouring green coloring on it."

"You wouldn't have put up with it—would you?" I was trying to get a rise out of her.

She didn't take the bait, but she did glare at me. "And, we can walk around and hold hands."

"Really?" I said.

"Yes, really. Nobody will see us."

"Everybody will see us. There's tons of people there."

"Yeah, but nobody we know."

"It doesn't matter if anybody knows you because it doesn't mean anything to you if someone sees us."

"It does mean something, you asshole."

"Whatever," I say. I turn around in Bobby Travis' body shop. He sees us, gives one of those loud whistles, and I have to stop. He's walking over, and Doris is sticking her head out of the window.

"Hey, Bobby," she says.

"Hey, Doris, how are you doing?" He bends down and peeps in to see me. "How's it going, man?"

"Good, Bobby, just working and playing." Doris laughs and looks from me to Bobby.

"Yeah, me, too. Congratulations, Kyle."

"Thanks, I guess." Me and Bobby laugh at this, but Doris starts talking again.

"Bobby, what are you up to this weekend?"

"Nothing really, I'm supposed to help Daddy with his car, probably drink a few beers with him. He's bringing it over first thing on Saturday."

"Maybe I'll come by?"

"Yeah, if you want. There's always a beer with your name on it, Doris."

"We got to go. See you, Bobby." That Bobby can be a son-of-a-bitch sometimes.

"Bye," Doris says.

If you walk far enough on Tambri's property, you'll run into the Lilly River. It's not very wide, but it is big enough to be called a river, and sometimes I'll go out there and fish. I usually don't catch a whole lot; it's really more about sitting there and listening to the river. If I'm by myself, I'll just doze off with my sunglasses on and my hands resting under my head for a pillow.

"That fish is not big enough to keep," Tambri said one time when we were sitting there in the grass and mud, right at the edge. There are trees and green all over the place. You look and it's like you're swimming in the color.

"Tambri, this is a fully grown catfish and it would be really delicious battered in corn meal and placed in a pan of popping grease," I said and pulled the hook out of its mouth; Tambri made a noise liked I'd yanked it out of her lip.

"That is a baby fish, and you can't keep it." She reached for it, and I held it above my head where she couldn't get to it.

"This carrot does not belong to you, little rabbit," I said, and I patted her on the head. She wasn't too crazy about that.

"I'm not stupid, and I'm not your little rabbit, and that is not your fish to keep." She was yelling now and trying to stand up and having a hard time with all the red mud under her feet. She would stand a little and slip, adjust her hands on the ground, move her feet closer to her butt, hoping that would make her more stable, and she'd stand a little and slip. She stopped struggling after a while and sat there, hands still on the ground, sticky mud oozing through the space between her fingers.

Doris would not have cared two flips about a fish.

"You're a thief," Tambri said.

"What?"

"Stealing that fish."

"Are you crazy?"

"What? Just because I don't go along with something that comes out of your mouth, I'm crazy? Have I got this straight?" She was really angry then, apparently angry enough to right herself up off the ground without even using her hands for support. She stood over me—I was still holding the slimy fish as it dripped above my head. The three of us were rungs on a ladder, Tambri, the fish, and then me at the bottom. If anybody had seen us, which I think the people living across on the other side of the lake probably did, they would have thought we had lost it.

She tried to take the fish out of my hand; I held on.

"Stop it, you're going to hurt it," she said.

"It is a fish with the brain the size of a flea, and it doesn't feel anything. And just so you know, a flea doesn't feel anything either." I have no idea why I was pushing the fish thing; maybe it was because I'd never seen her upset before, not angry anyway.

She let go and shoved me in the side with her foot; me and the fish tumbled into the cold lake, and I let go.

We're pulling into Doris' driveway.

"Wait," she says, and I stop the car. She gets out and picks up a yellow super-soaker gun and tosses it in the yard with all the other scattered toys. The kids are with their dad this week.

I keep the car running and sit here.

She stares at me, waiting. "What are you doing?" she says.

"I don't know," I say through the windshield. She doesn't understand me and comes back to my side of the car.

"What are you doing?" she says again. I guess she thinks I didn't hear her the first time.

"Just sitting here looking at all your kids' toys."

She glances at the yard like she hadn't noticed all the toys were there.

"Yeah, so what?" she says.

"I don't know," I say.

"Are you coming inside or what?"

"I'm not sure."

"Is that right? Let me tell you, you better get out of there and fast if you want to come inside my house again. You understand me?"

I look at her and don't say anything back.

"Bobby would be okay with coming over." She's got one hand on her hip and her other hand is clenched. "I don't have to be on your timetable. We can end this right now."

Do I want to end this?

"Like you're going to stop wanting me after nineteen days. What's going to happen? Are you going to change into somebody that doesn't enjoy touching me? Is that how it's going to work?"

I don't know.

"We're done. If you don't come into this house in one minute, we are through." She hesitates, still standing on her broken concrete driveway. She stares at me, turns around and stomps her way to the front door. She's stopping a minute to find her keys in her big orange purse and unlock the door. This breaks the effect a little, and it's not quite as dramatic as she wants.

I listen to the car running and her cussing me in the house. I roll up the windows, and turn on the radio—it's still on 99.4 where she left it.

The first time I stayed at Tambri's, I kept all my clothes on except my belt and my shoes, and I felt her breathing on my chest as she fell asleep across me. Nothing happened and I didn't want it to happen, not yet. I listened and hoped that she wouldn't stop wanting me there, and I was afraid to move.

What a big sucker, huh? Not sleeping all night, not wanting to wake her up. If Doris could have only seen me, she wouldn't have recognized the man in the bed.

When she did wake up early, I kept my eyes closed. She was quiet, and I listened as she turned the shower on and moved under the water. I opened my eyes and looked out the window into the pasture. I got up and left with my shoes and my belt in my hands at 6:45.

I knocked on Doris' door at 7:15.

Three songs have played, and I'm still in the car. My time's been up for quite a while, and I haven't left yet. The next-door neighbors have a sprinkler going over their little plot of grass. I turn the radio off to listen for Doris.

I don't hear anything; I roll my window down. Nothing. I turn the car off. The house is quiet, and I don't see her moving in the front window or any of the other windows that I search.

The decision's been made for me. I turn the car on and right before I pull out, she's holding the door open, standing in the frame.

A Snake or a Spider

My damp swimsuit sticks to me under my shorts and T-shirt. The water drained all my strength, and I imagine it floats in the lake somewhere. I stretch my arms toward the dash, and my limbs feel like molded jelly. Kyle moves the steering wheel with a steady rhythm, and we ride with the windows down. The warm breeze plays at my hair making it spiral and twist as it touches my face.

Kyle focuses on me with his dark brown eyes, and it seems that he cares for me. It was his idea that we go to the lake today. He said it was for me: a day of learning to relax. He wants good things for me. He's proven that with how he helps me with losing Sammy. Some people would say that fourteen years is long enough to suffer the death of a child and that I should move on.

No, I say. I don't have to move anywhere.

Kyle lets me talk when it overwhelms me. Most people just couldn't sit there, saying nothing. Everybody wants to offer comfort, encouraging words, something, but Kyle stays quiet, listening.

"Are you going to sleep?" he says as he shifts his eyes back to the road.

"I'm thinking about it." We're almost home so there isn't really time for sleep. I adjust myself in the seat, putting my hands under my butt and pushing myself up. I slide my hands out from under, and there's something weird brushing against my fingers.

"What is that?" I say, under my breath, as I pull my hand out quick and shift away from it. It gives me the creeps, and I really don't want to touch it. I purse my lips, determined to see what it is, as I pull it from the crease of the seat.

It's a hairnet, a black hairnet, still strange, but not as gross as it could have been. God, I'm glad it wasn't a spider web.

"What is it?" Kyle says, smiling, the skin puckering at the corners of his eyes. He's laughing at me for squirming around and making noises.

I place the hairnet on my index finger, letting it hang like a limp flag. I move my hand so that Kyle can get a better look at what I've found.

"Kyle, where did this come from?" I say. Did some idiot toss it aside after working at McDonald's, and it landed in the car? Maybe the person purposely threw it in the car, thinking it was funny. What's wrong with people?

Kyle looks over at what's in my hand and jerks his head back toward the road.

"I don't know what that is," he says, staring at the bumper of the car in front of us.

It's a hairnet, and I didn't ask him what it was. I asked where it came from, not thinking that he would really know.

"It's a hairnet," I say, and I am awake now. My stomach tightens with nausea.

"I see," he says, without turning to look at it again. His jaw clenches, and it's as if he thinks of the hairnet as a snake or a spider, something that should be squashed underfoot and forgotten.

I need to prove to him that it's just a hairnet. I put it on my head.

"Look, Kyle. I'm a lunchroom lady." I make a snorting sound and pretend to plop food onto invisible trays.

He looks over. "Take that off," he says. "You don't know where it's been."

Do you? I slide it off my head and feel the strangeness of it in my hand. I turn it over, squishing it with my fingers, and I think that a spider web would have been better for me. I tug at one section of the netting, pulling hard at the fibers. It can't give anymore, and it breaks between my fingers. I move to the next area and stretch the nylon cord until I hear the snap. I go from opening to opening, straining to shred this thing that Kyle knows nothing about. My fingers are raw, etched with lines from the thread. My pulse is in my fingertips, thumping, like something in a cartoon.

We turn into our driveway, and Kyle hasn't looked over at what's in my hand since I showed it to him.

"I'm going to throw this away," I say, shoving the remains of the hairnet in front of Kyle's face.

"Good," he says, "no telling where it came from." He takes his time getting out of the car. He's calmed himself down, and he walks to our door.

Did he act strange? Did it seem like he found the thing revolting?

I walk to the green plastic trash can that Kyle rolls out to the edge of the road every Thursday. I stare at the container having no intention of throwing away the balled up mess in my hand. Has Kyle tossed any other secrets away? I want to open the lid and rummage through the garbage like a raccoon. I'm not going to do it, though. Nobody wants to be a crazy woman. Is there someone who could test this thing for DNA like they do on T.V.? God, that's worse than considering going through the trash.

Damn it, Kyle, look what you've done.

I walk to my car, open the door, and put the evidence in my glove box. Why? I don't know. My strength has come back to me, and I slam the door closed. Kyle heard it, but he won't ask about it.

Who is this woman that for whatever reason wears a hairnet? She sounds glamorous.

∽

My insides are twisted with this doubt that's slipped in. I haven't said anything to Kyle. I've gone back to my car twice and stared at the black mass that seems to get bigger each time I open the glove box.

This sick gut of mine tells me there is something going on, but I'm not sure. I've thought about just asking Kyle. But if there isn't anything to this, what will that do to us? Either way, he's going to say, "There is nobody else, Tambri." My only choice, and I've thought about this, is to show Kyle that I trust him.

"Honey, are you almost finished?" I say.

We had a bad storm last night, and Kyle's been cutting the larger limbs that fell from the trees into more moveable pieces. He's been working ever since he got home. I've been waiting for an opportunity to come out here and talk to him.

"Yeah, I'm just putting the saw up," he says and he closes the door to the shed. "You look nice," he says, glancing at me starting with my shoes, working his way up, finally stopping at my face. "Are you going somewhere?"

"How would you like me to take you to dinner?" I say, and touch his sleeve.

"Tonight, now?"

"Yeah, I was thinking pizza and pasta."

"Monaco's?" he says, and he allows a smile to edge its way into his features, and the relief is apparent. "That sounds great to me, Tambri."

We walk side by side to the house, dead leaves crunching under our feet.

"I'll drive us in my car. I'll be your chauffeur, sir, for this evening's activities." I do a little bow toward Kyle.

"Fine by me," he says, chuckling at his good fortune. "I need to take a shower."

"Yes, you do, mister. Take your time; we're not in a hurry."

"Okay," he says, and kisses me on the cheek.

Is this the right thing to do? I don't know, but it's what came to me last night when I was lying in bed with Kyle deep in sleep next to me.

I'm patient sitting on the couch, almost holding my breath with abdomen muscles pulled tight and my back straight.

"Ready, Tambri," Kyle says as he comes up the hallway.

"Me, too," I say, but I wonder if I am.

We sit and chat and eat. Kyle is friendly to our waitress like he always is. That's something that I first liked about him. Everyone is on the same level for Kyle; no one is better or worse than anyone else.

The young waitress blushes as Kyle asks her about herself.

"Is this your main job," he says smiling at her, making her feel more comfortable.

"I go to school during the day."

"Where?" he says.

"Habersham Technical College. I'm going to be an X-Ray Technician."

"That's where Tambri went," Kyle says, and he pulls me in.

"Yeah?" the girl says, looking at me for support that she's made the right choice with her life.

"Yes, I'm a phlebotomist. I've been one for sixteen years now."

"You can make a good living at that," she says, approving of my choice.

"I think you'll enjoy being a tech," I say, wanting to give her the same approval. She's maybe twenty years old, and so unsure of everything.

She beams. "Listen, my name is Lisa. If you need anything, just let me know."

"Do you have extra cheese?" I say.

"Yes, I'll bring it right to you. I love it on my pasta, too."

"Thank you," Kyle and I both say.

Lisa rushes to the kitchen and hurries back with the cheese grater, loading Kyle and me up with a mound each. Lisa almost does a curtsy before she leaves the table. Kyle and I smile at each other, knowing how it feels to be that unsure.

"Tambri, I'm glad you had this idea. This is delicious," he says and laps up a noodle from his plate.

We laugh, and talk, and eat, and add more butter to our bread, and salt to our food. We drink wine and, we sit, melting farther into our chairs until we're stuffed.

"I ate too much, Tambri," Kyle says, sitting in the passenger seat with his eyes closed, stretching his arms above his head. I drive us home.

The radio is turned up just enough to be heard and someone is talking, but I can't understand what she's saying. I press the radio off, happy for the silence. I need to ask Kyle something.

"Kyle, there's some gum in the glove box, can you hand me a piece?"

He slowly opens his eyes, leans forward and pushes the button. The door of the box flops open, and the light pours out of the little space.

"What is this, Tambri?" he says and there is anger in his voice.

I stare at the road.

"Answer me. What is this?" His jaw is clenched as he talks. From the corner of my eye, I see that he is holding the tangled threads. He slams the button to let the window down, and throws the hairnet out.

"I don't want to talk anymore about this, Tambri," he says.

We weren't talking about it, Kyle.

❧

"That looks good on you," Kyle says. He sits on the bed watching me get ready.

I put on my earrings, looking in the mirror and catching the shine of the silver on my neck as I move back and forth, pretending to care how this dress looks. The glint of the chain around my throat seems out of place. From what's inside me, it's absurd to wear anything that shines.

I walk to the closet looking for my shoes. Under flip flops, tennis shoes, and a couple of dropped hangers are my pair of black pumps. I pick them up and turn around.

Kyle is in front of me. I stare at him blankly. He moves closer, and I backup into the closet, against the clothes. He rests his hands on the rod behind me, placing them on either side of my head. I bend down trying to slip under his elbow, but he is too fast. He stops me with his left hand, holding my shoulder and rubbing it at the same time. My shoes dangle from my hand.

He closes his eyes and rubs his cheek along the side of my face. "You smell sweet, too," he says. I lean back from him, long sleeves of shirts wrapping around me. He thinks if I let him put his hands on me, if I let him have me, I'll surrender to his way of things.

"It's because I just took a shower."

"It's too much for one man to take."

You're too much for one woman to take, aren't you?

"You need to get dressed, too," I say, but he just stands there looking down at me, coming closer, as if he's about to kiss me. I slap the bottom of my shoes on top of his arm.

Dirty soles on his skin break the mood. He lets go of the bar behind me, and I move around out of the dark closet, into the room.

This is his aunt's wedding that we're going to, and he's the one that wants to mess around and make us late. It's not going to happen.

Fourth marriage, and I still don't know all the things that men can do. And this is probably the one that I should have thought about the most. They can pull you through a ringer, turning the crank and telling you how sweet you smell at the same time.

I watch Kyle put on his pants.

"You know she's younger than me," he says.

My insides jump.

"Who?" I say, leaning down to brush off the bottom of my bare feet. I slide into my shoes and stand up to brace myself.

"My aunt. My grandparents had another kid after I was born. Two more kids. I have two aunts younger than me."

I turn away from him inspecting my clothes in the mirror one last time. I take a deep breath. I hope that he can't tell that I'm flustered.

Have any of my ex-husbands ever cheated on me? I'm sure of one and three. Daniel and Clay. Not so sure about number two and very unsure about number four. I guess I'm luckier with odd numbers.

Thinking about it, the only way to be sure about a man is to hang under him day and night, watching everything he does.

As bad as this is right now, losing Sammy pained me more than anything else ever could. This is a cake walk, and I'm just waiting for the music to stop.

I remember my grandmother telling me about men.

"If a man gives you flowers more often than twice a year—you're in trouble."

Another one of hers was "always wash your swimsuit as soon as you take it off." I didn't pay attention to that one either.

"It's a magic trick without any magic. He'll put the pretty flowers with their bright colors and sugary fragrance in front of you to block your view of his dark heartedness."

"Really," I said, as I painted my nails a bright shade of pink, thinking that my grandmother could be so dramatic sometimes. I was about fifteen then, and I thought I knew more than anybody, especially an old woman that lived alone. How would she know?

I don't think I can put a number to the times Kyle's given me flowers since we've been married. There's too many.

❧

The bride wears lace. I've never worn lace, but Kyle's aunt looks beautiful in it. I hope she does better than me. Kyle is whispering to me as we sit back down on the wooden pews.

"I don't want to stay for the reception," he says. He keeps his face toward the bride and groom. No one else would know that he had said a word to me. Look how good he is at keeping secrets.

I ignore him. I want to see the church. It's a catholic church, and I've only been inside once. There's only a couple in town. This one and St. Christopher's on Hemlock Street.

I came to this church the Thanksgiving after Sammy died. I thought helping other people would help me. That's what people kept telling me anyway, especially Vickie. I always knew she was a good friend—I didn't know how much she cared about me until everything happened with Sammy.

"It will help your soul," she would say.

"What does that even mean?"

"Go to the church," she said. She said it at least ten times.

"You can go to the church and then you and Daniel can come over here for Thanksgiving dinner."

So, I went to the church.

I stood in the meeting hall at the very back handing out plates of food. The smell made me queasy. It didn't smell bad to anyone else, I don't think.

"Thank you, sugar," an older black lady said. She wore thick glasses, and her hair was tucked under a burgundy scarf. She didn't live on the street, but I could tell things were tight for her. Of course they had to be. She was picking up free Thanksgiving dinner at a church.

I watched her move to one of the round tables, watched as she said her prayer, watched as she ate without saying a word to anyone else sitting at her table. I hoped that she would show me something, teach me something that Vickie thought helping in church would force me to see. I felt sad for the lady; she had it rough in a different way. I didn't feel better.

I stopped staring at the woman and handed plates of food to a woman probably about my age at the time—mid-twenties, and her two children. I watched the three of them, too. They sat down and ate. Nothing more, just sat there and ate. Well, the mother would cut up the turkey for the youngest girl. I think the littlest girl was maybe four or so. I realized that I was angry with the woman. She looked at me a couple of times, and I would turn my face in another direction, but she knew that I was staring, and she couldn't understand why. Hell, I didn't know why for a little while.

I had no idea who she was; she'd never done anything to piss me off or anything. How could she have? And then I realized that no matter what other bad thing had happened to her, no matter how broke she was—she had her two daughters sitting beside her. She could feel the warmth of their bodies on either side of her; she could see the tangle of the smaller one's blonde hair, and I resented that woman more than anyone.

I left without seeing any other part of the church.

And now, Kyle wants to boss me and rush me out. He can forget it.

All the windows are stained glass, with Jesus on one window, Mary on another. The sun burns through the bright colors and the light breaks where the darker panes lay. It adds to the celebration for the couple standing timidly in front of the priest.

"I do," Kyle's soon-to-be uncle says. He is not a tall man, next to his bride with her heels on, heels that no one can see at the moment, he is a full inch shorter. He beams up at her, licking his lips after the words spill out.

"I do," she says.

I let my mind drift as they move over to the candles and light them with regular lighters. Red Bic lighters. I'm guessing that Kyle's aunt or uncle, or both, smoke. I stifle a giggle, and cough to cover it up. They each light one of the outside candles, and then together they light the middle candle. I look at Kyle to see if he's noticed the Bics. He's looking straight ahead, and he's grinding his teeth. What's going on with him?

The couple stands still in front of the candles waiting for something or someone that's taking more time than was planned. Finally, the sound of a lady singing comes from behind us. Everyone turns around to see a fifty-something lady singing "Ava Maria" from the balcony. Her voice is nice, soothing. I turn back around and just listen, closing my eyes and letting the music wash over me.

I open my eyes and realize that Kyle is facing forward, too. He's in an odd mood today, and I watch him from the corner of my eye. He scans the faces that look up, and he stops on one in particular. He glances at me, and I stay still like I haven't noticed that he was looking at me or anyone else.

I see the woman he sees.

Out of everyone in the room, we seem to be the only three not looking at the couple in the front of the church, or the singer at the back of the church. She, this woman, is looking at Kyle, and Kyle and I both are looking at her. The sick, dropping feeling is back in my stomach, but the look on Kyle's face seems normal, now. He looks over at me and takes my hand, squeezing it as he looks at the couple. Almost as if he's saying to me, "Remember when we got married, honey?"

The song ends, and the couple and everyone else shifts back to where they were before it began.

It's official now.

"You may kiss the bride," the priest says. He raises his hands for everyone to rise. The couple turn, hesitating for one second before they begin walking toward the exit of the church.

Kyle's aunt smiles like she's beaten all odds and won the lottery; she holds her husband's hand, but it looks like that isn't enough for her. She crosses her right hand over her body, still holding the bouquet, and places that hand on his left hand. The red and pink roses have consumed their hands. "Look at her leaning on him, already," most people say to themselves. I can see it in the way the lady on the fourth row nods her head as they walk past her.

I know better.

If Kyle's aunt could, she'd put him up in seclusion somewhere. She'd be the only one to sleep with him. She'd make sure of it. At least she knows for right this minute he's not doing anything with anyone else. This is a public place. A church. She and all these people would stop him.

It's the secret places and times when he is away that scare her.

"Did you hear what I said, Tambri?" Kyle's talking again, still wanting me to give in and go home.

"This is a catholic church, Kyle. They'll be wine, women, and song. You like those—don't you?"

"What are you talking about?"

"We're staying." I walk toward the reception hall.

"I don't want to."

"If you want, you can go on home. Someone will give me a ride."

That shuts him up. He follows me as we move along with all the people.

"Are you sure you want to stay and eat all this finger food crap?"

"You liked it at our wedding," I say, hurrying forward, breaking away from him.

The reception hall sits below the church. I take the stairs and walk in to the mostly dingy white room that I've seen once before. It's different this time with about ten or twelve round tables covered with white paper tablecloths that hang to the floor. Each table contains a clear vase that holds the same items as Kyle's aunt's bouquet: red and pink roses.

A few silver balloons are scattered around the room, tied to the backs of chairs. There aren't quite enough balloons to fill the space, and some of them strain against the pull of the black metal fans that rotate above.

I stand in the middle of the room pretty much by myself, and I feel silly and obvious. I meander to the outer edges of the room, where almost everyone else is. A few of the brave souls are lining up at the buffet while everyone else looks sheepish, not wanting to appear over eager. Most people are paired up, or have kids, or stand with friends. Kyle is standing in the corner by himself. Yes, you have been bad, Kyle. Stand there, and take your punishment.

I search for someone else I know. I don't want to wimp out and leave because I'm uncomfortable. I see someone with a glass of red wine. Maybe that would help me feel a little less foolish.

I move to the table with the drinks. I pick up a glass and take a small sip. The wine is warm; it heats the lining of my throat and melts the nausea in my stomach. Just holding the glass with the long stem gives me some confidence to stand here a few more minutes.

There's a guy I know. He's a patient of Dr. Kimberly, my boss. I have to stop myself from running to him. I make an effort to walk toward him, trying to think of his name. What is his name? I should know it. Richard, Rodney...

something with an R. I really wish I could think of it before he turns around.

And he's turning around, and I still can't remember.

"Hey there," he says to me, "do you have a request before I get started?" He doesn't remember me, but he doesn't seem opposed to talking to me.

"D.J. Ronald" it says on the front of his station that he's set up. Yep, that's his name. I'm glad there's a sign.

"Ronald, do you remember me?"

He looks at me more focused. "Yes," he says. "You took some of my blood. That's okay though, I've been getting along just fine without it."

"Yes," I say, and laugh at his joke. I've never been so happy to be recognized by someone. "In case you don't remember, my name is Tambri."

"I'm not sure I ever knew what it was," he says. "I don't care that much about needles. I try to get in and out as quick as I can when it comes to that."

"Most people feel the same way."

"It's good talking to you, Tambri. I better get started."

"Good to see you, too." Either the wine that I've been gulping or Ronald has put me in a better frame of mind.

I linger at Ronald's table watching as he slips in CD's and adjusts various buttons.

The music starts, and it's a slow one. It's an old Ray Charles song. *Come Rain or Come Shine.* Beautiful.

I wander around the room, watching people, softly singing the song to myself. There's a tall fountain with some kind of foamy drink coming out of it. From the color, I'm guessing it's orange sherbet.

There's applause, and the bride and groom walk in.

"Announcing Mr. and Mrs. Jesup Stevens!" Ronald says. They head straight for the dance floor. She kisses him lightly on the lips as he wraps his arm around her back. Everyone seems relieved that they're finally here, and the party can begin.

I'm standing by the four-tier bride's cake. It looks like it came from Cynthia's Bakery downtown. Cynthia always decorates with the smallest little flowers.

There's a girl of about five standing on the other side of the cake, and she's peeping around at me. I give her a wave with my free hand. She waves back.

"Hey," she says.

"Hey," I say back.

"You should try the icing," she says. She holds her index finger out for me to see. There's a big clump of icing setting on it. She sticks her finger in her mouth.

"It's good," she says and shows me her sugar-covered teeth.

"No thanks," I say, and I can't help but laugh. She disappears around the cake again, and I have no doubt that her finger is stuck in the icing.

Everyone is dancing now to a fast song. The small parquet floor is almost full. I guess some of the folks were dying to get out there. What else is there to do, though, besides standing around staring at people, eating this crappy finger food, or just surrendering and leaving?

I'm taking my shoes off; they hurt, and I can't dance in them. I pull them off with my left hand and tuck them under the cake table. The little girl watches me.

"I'll take care of them for you," she says.

"Thank you," I say and turn back to her to give her a thumbs up as I walk to the dance floor.

There's about four or five women dancing all together, and they look friendly and willing to take one more. I smile and try to gesture with my shoulders asking, "Can I join?" One of the ladies is already half lit.

"Come on in," she says motioning with her arm. She's tall and big. She's probably late fifties, early sixties. She may be the lady that was singing earlier. She is bopping back and forth, and her big dress moves the opposite direction that her body moves, as if it's trying to catch up. Her shoes are off, too, and she taps the ball of each foot on the floor, feeling the beat and kicking the hell out of it.

I move a little, and I try to remember the last time I danced. I can't. I mean I can remember dancing—I just don't remember when the last time was. I wonder if I can even do this. I'm still holding what's left of my glass of wine. The big lady notices it the same time I do.

"Drink it down, honey." She laughs, and shakes her head, and does a spin in front of me.

I drink until it's all gone, and now I don't have to worry about dancing with a glass of wine. The lady takes it from me and sets it gently on the table next to the dance floor. When she turns back around, I'm dancing.

I've forgotten what this feels like, to move for no reason except to dance. I'm off the beat, I can tell. God, I hate people that dance and aren't with the beat. I close my eyes trying to focus on the song that Ronald's playing. My arms and legs seem to be fighting with each other, and I don't know what the hell my middle is doing. I need to slow down and breathe.

I stand still and close my eyes. I listen, and listen, and listen. I wonder how long I've been standing here with my eyes closed, now. I don't care—finding the beat is more important than what these people think.

I start to move again, and it's like the thump of Ronald's song is under my arms, under my feet, moving them without me pushing them to move. I laugh and open my eyes hoping for the big lady's approval. Kyle is standing in front of me.

He puts his hand on my cheek, and I keep dancing. He wants me to stop, but I won't.

"Dance with me," I say. I watch as he thinks about what he should do next. He sticks his hands in his pockets.

"Tambri, I don't know how to dance." He's such a liar.

"Okay, then don't." I twirl around trying to imitate the big lady's move. I look down and see Kyle's feet moving on the floor. Shuffling is a better word. One foot forward and back, then the other foot forward and back. God, I want to laugh, but he is trying so hard.

I glance up to his arms, and they are moving in the motion of a train. I watch his face, and he's almost biting his lip from all the concentration.

Would a man do this if he was cheating on his wife?

He looks back at me and smiles and moves his arms faster. It looks like he's picking up speed, pulling out of the station.

"All aboard," I say and copy what he's doing. We bust out laughing.

"Choo-Choo," Kyle says and moves away from me shaking his caboose.

The big lady joins in. "Choo-Choo," she says.

This feels good. My cheeks burn from the alcohol and the dancing, and I can feel sweat sliding down the back of my neck to my shoulder blades. Kyle and I dance and dance, until we're both winded, and aching from laughing.

Enough fun. The big lady looks like she's nowhere near stopping; and I wave goodbye to her as she starts up with another song.

Kyle and I step off the floor together. The little girl must have been watching the whole time because she's running over to me with my shoes.

"I kept them safe," she says, and I take them from her feeling her sticky fingers touch mine.

"You are sweet," I say, watching as she giggles and runs back to the cake.

I slide my shoes on, smiling at the thought of the little girl. Kyle and I sit at a table full of dirty dishes.

"What do you want to drink, honey?" he says as he stands up. I turn away from him to watch all the dancers.

"As long as it's cold, I'll drink it." I look back at him, and I can see that he's hot and sweaty.

He turns, and there is a look of recognition that comes over his face. The same look that he had for the woman in the church. The same kind of expression on Ronald's face when he realized that he knew me.

Now it's gone, but I know that I saw it. My arms become chilled as the breeze from the fans cool the sweat on my skin. I glance in the direction that Kyle was looking in. There she is, the same woman from before.

"Here you go," Kyle says as he hands me a plastic glass of ice water. He blocks my view and continues to stand in front of me. "Thank you," I say to him. It almost comes out in a whisper, and I rise from my chair and move around him, avoiding the reach of his arm.

She's moved from where she was standing. I search the room, through all the people, and it seems like everything has slowed in front of me. I know that I only have to look a little closer, and she'll show herself to me. All I have to do is focus, and she'll appear.

The woman in the middle. I haven't thought about what she might look like, and I only got a quick glimpse of her round face and dark hair before. But there she is. Tight dress, lots of makeup, and lots of extra pounds. Lots of extra pounds.

Do you have to look the part? Don't you have any originality in your bones? I want to yell these things to her, but I don't. I just stare at her, and I know that Kyle is staring at me.

"You want to dance, again?" he says in my ear. It sounds like some kind of plea. Please, please, dance with me, Tambri.

"No, I don't want to dance with you anymore," I say. I don't move my gaze from this woman that Kyle obviously knows. Kyle's sweating more now than when we were dancing.

She's looking at me, almost daring me, but to do what? To call her what she is in the gathering hall of a catholic church. No thanks, hairnet-wearing glamour girl.

"Kyle, I think I'm ready to go, honey." He doesn't have to know for sure about what I've figured out. That's the character of men like Kyle—they're always so hopeful. Hopeful that the other woman will be okay with being just that. Hopeful that his wife will always be ignorant to what he is doing when she isn't around.

"Whatever you say," Kyle says, and he puts his hand on the lower part of my back and leads me to the door. He so desperately wants to turn his attention to her to see what she is doing, to see how she is doing.

※

My feet are covered, but they're still cold. It's my fault. I walked around the house again before bed without shoes. It's not really my feet, but my toes. They feel like ice. I lie on my back and wriggle them trying to get some circulation going.

Kyle lies beside me with his back facing me. I can tell he's not asleep by the way he's breathing. He's pretending to be asleep, making his breath sound deep, but it's just too shallow, and I can tell. I can see a lot of things about him now.

Maybe I should have known sooner. I've been cheated enough in my life. I would think I would get some kind of feeling sooner than I did, something in my stomach, or under my skin, or in my head. Somewhere, but that doesn't matter. I know now, and it's over and done with. Kyle just doesn't know it, yet.

But he sure as hell is lying there wondering. "Does she know?" is what he's thinking. Over and over. Lie there and wonder, Buddy.

God, my toes are almost numb. I bend my knees, and stomp my feet up and down on the bed, making the covers rise and fall around my legs.

Kyle doesn't move. Still wondering, huh Kyle?

I stomp some more, no feeling in my toes, yet, and nothing from Kyle's side of the bed. I laugh out loud at how ridiculous this is.

Enough.

I turn over to face his back, pull my knees toward my chest, like I'm about to do a jackknife into a pool, and stick my frozen toes into the pit of his back. He flies out of the bed, sucking in air, "Son-of-a-bitch, Tambri," rolling off his tongue.

Yes, Kyle. Son-of-a-bitch.

Vickie's Husband

How long is someone supposed to mourn? I don't know. I guess no one ever gets over the death of a child, especially when he was so little, already walking and talking. The potential of the child is just beginning to show through. Personality's there.

"Tambri, you have to move on," my wife will say. This is a common conversation. I don't know why Vickie thinks she can fix Tambri.

I love Tambri like she's my little sister, I really do, but this has been going on for a long time. I usually don't say anything, though.

I don't want to come across as callous; I'm not that at all. God knows I miss Sammy, too. He was only four years old and bright as the noon sun.

I keep all these thoughts to myself. Vickie's on a mission when it comes to Tambri. I'm just the quiet guy that sits at the table with his wife and her best friend, and listens as they do most of the talking.

"Let's don't talk about that," Tambri says. See, she's even getting tired of Vickie trying to make everything better.

The three of us sit around a table at the diner on Highway 49. They have the best fried onions here.

"How are things at work?" Tambri says, looking at me.

"Fine, just busy, which is good," I say and laugh a little. I take a sip of tea.

Vickie glances over at me like she's saying, "Shut-up and let me talk to her."

"Maybe you should take some classes. You know they say using your hands is good for a distraction."

"What kind of class are you thinking about?" Tambri says. She looks over at me for help. I shrug my shoulders.

"I don't know, Tambri," Vickie says. "I can't tell you every-thing. Sewing, maybe."

"Nope," Tambri says.

"Cross-stitch."

"Nope."

"What about some kind of instrument? Guitar."

"Nope," Tambri says, and she punches me in the side to let me know she's just messing with Vickie. I wish she wouldn't do that; it just gets Vickie going. I give Tambri a halfway smile, letting her know I'm in on the game.

Vickie sees the whole thing.

"What about the class they call kiss my ass, honey?" Vickie says, but she's not looking at Tambri, she's looking at me. I'm the one that always catches hell. I lift my hands up in front of me. "What," I signal to Vickie.

"Don't you even start," she says to me. I fold my arms across my chest and try to stay out of the way.

"Don't be mad with him, Vickie. I'm the one that started it."

"Yeah, but he knows better. He's the one that sleeps in the same bed with me." She gives me one last eat-shit look.

I scan the laminated menu.

And they continue without me. Vickie trying to talk Tambri into some kind of lesson that Tambri doesn't want to take, and Tambri saying "no" to every one of them. Sometimes when their conversations get this heated, they forget I'm sitting here.

I get bored with it. I want to talk about something else. I want to talk more about what happened with me today. I could tell them about the guy that cussed me out over the phone because he didn't like the way I did his taxes. The fact was he didn't want to pay the taxes he owed. The asshole ended up hanging up on me. I placed the receiver back down on its cradle and took a deep breath, picked up my pencil and went back to work.

The trickiness of Tambri is that she can sit at a table in a restaurant and act like she's okay. She'll laugh and joke, just like everybody else. She puts on this face for other people, and that includes me and Vickie, sometimes.

But then, something will trigger something else, and all of a sudden everything turns into a hail storm.

Tambri called the house the other night at 1:30 in the morning. 1:30 in the morning. Vickie woke up and grabbed the phone. It's always on her side of the bed for just such an occasion.

"Okay, okay," she said. "We'll be right there, just hang on, we'll be right there."

"She's upset," she said, and hung up the phone.

I figured as much. "What happened?" I said.

"She's upset, that's all I know." It always sounds like she's angry with me. I don't understand it, and I don't know what to do about it.

"She still has his room the same, you know," she said.

"I know."

"Every Saturday when I go over to her house to help her clean, I peek in his room. It's always the same."

"I know," I said.

"She won't even let me in there. I've asked her if it needs to be cleaned. She always says, 'No, leave it alone, Vickie.'"

Every time my wife says that I want to yell, "Then, leave it alone. Leave Tambri alone. Let her work through it whatever crazy way she wants to work through it." But, I don't.

What good would it do anyway?

Vickie glanced at me for reassurance. I took her hand and smiled at her as we got in the car at 1:30 in the morning to drive over to Tambri's house.

"It's been so many years," she said almost crying, but holding the tears off because she didn't want Tambri to see.

So many husbands, too, I thought. I know that's smartass, but I get so tired of it.

"This is all so wrong," Vickie said.

"Yes, it is," I said, but I didn't mean it like Vickie thought. It's wrong that Vickie keeps doing what she feels she has to do for Tambri. If Vickie had known for a second what I thought, she might have pushed me out of the car and drove over there by herself.

"You know, she'll be okay, Vickie," I said. I couldn't believe that I had said it.

"You think so?" she said.

"Yes, of course, she needs to be by herself to figure out how to work through this herself."

"Are you kidding me? That's what you meant? I thought you meant she would be okay in general."

Then she pushed the top of my arm.

"You didn't hear her on the phone. You don't know her like I do."

Of course, I don't, I thought. No one knows her like you do, not even God.

I continued to drive to Tambri's.

"I'm sorry," I said. "We need to check on her."

"Damn right, we do."

When we got there, Tambri was a mess. Her eyes were swollen and her hair looked like she'd been twirling different pieces of it through her fingers.

"I'm sorry I called," Tambri said looking at me. Sometimes I think she knows what I'm thinking; then I end up feeling guilty.

"No, it's fine, Tambri," I said, "besides, you know Vickie, she is a loyal friend. And the loyal friend has a loyal husband that follows her wherever she goes." What the hell did that even mean?

"Tambri, I'm going to make you some hot tea. That'll soothe your nerves," Vickie said.

"I'll make it," I said. "You go talk with Tambri."

They left me alone in the kitchen making tea in the middle of the night. I caught bits and pieces of the words. At certain points, Tambri seemed to be whimpering.

That bothered me. I wanted to do something to help, but I couldn't think of a single thing. So, I finished making two cups of tea, one for Tambri and one for Vickie, and I waited until I didn't hear anything that sounded like crying, and I eased into Tambri's bedroom.

Vickie was rocking Tambri against her shoulder, and Tambri looked like she was almost asleep.

I put the tea on the bedside table and slid back out.

I went to the car and got my laptop, brought it back in, and sat in the living room surfing, while Vickie consoled Tambri. I was just the driver, waiting for my fare.

We got back home about 3:30. I couldn't sleep, so I did some work, and I finally went to bed about 4:30. I got up at 6:30, not a lot of sleep for an accountant, not a lot of sleep for anybody.

It's almost like we have this baby that lives six-and-a-half miles from us. When she cries, we have to run to her every time. Every time.

We've cancelled two vacations. On one I lost the deposit of a thousand bucks. I'm not made out of money. I tried to tell Vickie that one time, and she ignored me. I know that she heard me. It's as if whatever it takes, she'll do it for Tambri.

Isn't that statement supposed to end with my name? Isn't it the husband that the wife should do anything for, because I do absolutely everything for Vickie. That includes taking her to Tambri's in the middle of the night. That includes listening to her talk about how much she agonizes over Tambri.

I listen, I cajole, I worry about how long Vickie can do this. I wonder how long we can do this.

∽

I've just left Vickie in the house. We had a fight; nobody has to guess what it was about. We rarely argue. Most of the time I think it's just not worth it. I don't know. Something just blew inside me this time.

I walk around and around the block. I change directions a couple of times and go the other way. I head back toward our front door.

Vickie's standing on the brick steps watching me walk up.

"Don't do that again," she says crying into her hands. "I was worried about you. You've been gone for over an hour."

I was? I didn't realize it had been that long.

"I'm sorry, baby. I didn't mean to make you anxious."

"No, you're right. I do run to Tambri too much. I do try to fix everything."

Really? I move my fingertips along the metal of the railing.

"I promise I'll do better."

"You don't have to promise something like that."

"Yes, I do. I never thought about the way that you put it. I should make you the top priority in my life. Our marriage is the number one thing."

"Okay," I say, "stop crying." I put my arm around her shoulder and lead her inside. It's not often that she's like this. I'm not used to it.

"Do you want a drink?" I ask her. I know I need one.

"Yeah, that sounds like a good idea." She's calmed down some, and she's wiping her eyes with the sleeve of her shirt. Her hands shake a little.

Neither one of us says anything while I make the drinks. Jack and Coke, it's both our favorite.

I hand her the drink, and she puts it up to her forehead.

"I cried like an idiot, and now I have a headache," she says, laughing at herself.

"You're not an idiot. I shouldn't have been so loud. I shouldn't have said so much."

"You have to. You might explode if you don't." We laugh at that.

"And that wouldn't be a pretty sight," I say.

I grab her hand and swing our arms back and forth.

"It's just I don't know what to do sometimes," she says.

"Me, too."

"When Tambri calls, I just don't know how to say no. You know what I mean?"

"Yes, I do know what you mean." I take a sip of my drink and release her hand.

"How can you say no to someone who has lost their baby boy?"

"We'll figure this out together," I say.

"I just worry so much about her."

I take another sip.

"I stay awake sometimes and wonder that she might do something to herself."

I drop my head and study the strands of the carpet.

"She called while you were gone."

"Did you tell her about our fight?"

"No, of course not, that's between you and me." She smiles at me.

"Good." I smile back at her. "What did you talk about?"

"Different things."

"Like what."

"You know, the usual. She said her day was tough at work. I talked about my day and how much money I made in tips at the shop."

"How much did you make?"

"Around sixty-five dollars. One lady, who I thought wasn't going to tip me anything because she didn't talk the entire time I was working on her hair, gave me fifteen dollars."

"That's really good, Vickie. She must have liked the way you cut her hair."

"I guess so." She has a pleased look on her face. I like to see her like that.

"Then, Tambri was telling me about this eighteen-year-old kid that she had to draw blood from today. They think he might have some kind of cancer."

"That's awful, Vickie."

"Yeah, he made her think about Sammy, him being so close to the age that Sammy would have been. You understand that, don't you, honey?"

"Of course, I'm not a monster," I say.

"I told Tambri I'd bring her something over for dinner. I hope you don't mind? I'm afraid she won't eat at all, if I don't take something to her."

"Of course, we've got some of the chili left over."

"Yeah, that's what I was thinking I would take her."

"Do you want me to drive you?"

"No, you stay here and relax with your drink." She grabs the covered bowl of chili from the counter. I hadn't noticed it before now. She kisses me on the cheek.

"You know I love you," she says.

"I love you, too."

She walks out the front door and leaves me alone in the den drinking my Jack and Coke.

Injury

"When we get in here, help me look for that DVD," Vickie says.

"Okay, what's the name of it again?" I say.

Vickie has brought me to a new sporting goods store called *Sports and More*. Today is grand opening day, and we're walking through the parking lot. It's packed with cars. Vickie said they're giving away prizes, the biggest being a cruise.

"*Pummeling the Pounds*," Vickie says, and she smiles. She likes the name; she's putting her hopes of losing ten pounds in two weeks into that title. Not that she's going somewhere in two weeks. It's just how they're promoting it.

There's a red and black floating man by the front door. Air keeps catching him, and he bounces back up straight, and then almost hits the ground again. I know how you feel, I think as we walk past him.

Vickie always goes for this kind of stuff. I don't even think she needs to lose weight. My grandmother said that you shouldn't worry about such things. You may need the few extra pounds if you get sick or something. Vickie doesn't believe in that train of thought at all. She prefers to buy into what everyone else expects from her. I'm sure that includes me.

I lean on Vickie too much and too often. She never says anything, but shit, I get tired of me. I know she does.

The glass doors, that will only be this clean and shiny for today, slide open without much noise, and Vickie and I walk in. People are everywhere, and the lines are long. They're supposed to be having some pretty good sales, too.

"Where do you think the workout programs are?" Vickie says as she searches the signs.

Bright yellow and green signs hang from the ceiling. The white letters almost seem to move against the bright neon background. It's loud, the signs and the store. It's like Christmas.

"There they are," she says, and walks in the direction that she's pointing to.

I hope the DVD is here. It's sold out everywhere else. They've really been running the commercials.

There's energy and movement in this store. I see a woman in her late twenties trying on a pair of white Keds. She stands up and moves from one spot to another, lifting her feet, bending to touch her toes. It's funny to see how flexible she is. Maybe I should get a pair of Keds.

We're slowing down. An older lady, probably in her eighties, is walking with her grandson. She's holding his hand and neither one of them seem to be in any kind of hurry.

They're annoying Vickie because they're taking just enough of the aisle up to block her from getting by. Vickie's looking over at me now, rolling her eyes.

"Why don't they damn move?" is what she's saying.

I can see all the way to the back of the store. It almost has a warehouse feel to it. Everything echoes just a little, if you stop for a second and tune your ear just right.

"Make sure to register for our door prizes at the back of the store," the store manager says over the booming microphone. "Our grand prize is a cruise to Cozumel, Mexico!"

"Let's do that, Tambri," Vickie says. This kind of stuff makes her happy: buying a workout DVD and registering for something. She's always hopeful, even when it comes to me.

"There's the box to sign up for the cruise," she says, picking up speed to register, forgetting about her DVD. She rushes past two teenage boys who are a little off the main walkway to the right. They're practicing their swings with baseball bats. She gets their attention as she yells back to me. They turn and face her, both still feeling the grip of the bats and almost competing on how hard each can swing at the imaginary ball flying towards them.

"Vickie, here's the aisle with the DVD's," I say, pointing. She's out of earshot, and she's got only one thing on her mind right now. I'd better look for it. You never know, they may only have a few in stock. She's wanted this thing for a while now.

They have it. I pick it up, and turn it over to the back.

"Three times a week and you're in the best shape you've ever been in," Amber Donovan, Washington, D.C.

Amber's smiling big in her tight workout shorts and T-shirt. She does look in shape.

They have three left, but this one is Vickie's. I walk towards her, and it's like she can feel me looking at her because she turns around. I'm holding up the DVD pointing to it with my other hand, smiling at her, mouthing, "Here it is. Here it is."

She claps. From the side of my eye, I catch the movement of the two guys swinging, and the wind of one of the bats moves my hair. Vickie stops clapping, and her face falls.

My head rotates fast with a hard, sharp pain. My vision shifts, separating into two. My legs give way, and my knees buckle. Boom, skin and bones make contact with cement, and my body is jarred again as my knees hit the floor.

There's buzzing everywhere and it seems to be loudest on the right side of my brain. I cover my ears, but the constant noise won't go away. The pain runs through my nerves, and my torso sways. I have to stop myself from falling on my face. This hurts enough; I can't stand to hurt more. I balk against the forward direction my body seems intent on. I force my butt back, landing hard on my heels, eyes closed.

Everything is spinning, and I'm worried that I might fall to one side or the other. Something is bracing me. I open my eyes, turning to see two legs in ragged blue jeans, and a baseball bat hanging from a hand.

I lift my head as much as I can and see that it's one of the teenagers. The blow came from that bat. I stare at it, hoping to see where it might have given way, a small piece of splintered wood just to show that I had made an impact.

The boy, and that's all he is, just a big boy, is about to cry.

"I'm so sorry," he mouths over and over, but I can't really hear anything besides the buzzing. Everything is slowing down. Everyone's movements are off.

I feel bad for the boy. I'm sure I deserved it.

I want to bounce back up so that he can see that I'm okay, but my body refuses. I lean against him, and he holds me by the shoulder, securing me in place. I'm grateful for the anchor.

My hearing is coming back in pieces, but the pain is worse.

"Tambri, are you okay?" Vickie is running towards me and I think, don't run, I don't want you to fall, but there are no words coming out of my mouth.

"Oh, my God. Oh, my God," she says, and now everything is a flurry of people around me. I've been circled. There are people everywhere. Faces looking at me. I can't make out everything that's being said, but it's about me. I can feel their eyes on me. How can it not be about me?

Vickie searches my face, checking my pupils. "Tambri, follow my finger," she says.

I'm sorry, Vickie, I don't think I can. Why would you want me to?

I watch as someone pulls out a phone and dials with purpose. Good, get someone here to help me.

"Do you want to lie down?" Vickie says.

I shake my head. I don't want to lie on this dirty floor.

I watch the people looking down at me. I look through the cracks of their legs to find something that makes sense. I see the grandmother and the little boy walking towards us. I remember them from before. They aren't in a hurry. Everyone else seems frantic, but they seem to be the only ones I understand. They're on the same wavelength as me. I know them, but where do I know them from?

I blink and blink again, trying to focus on only them.

Vickie is in my face again.

"Tambri, let's ease you into this chair."

"Okay," I say, but my voice is so low I'm not sure if she can hear me. I'd forgotten she was here. I'm being lifted, mostly by my shoulders by Vickie, the boy, and maybe two other people. One feels like a child's little hands.

I close my eyes as I sit, trying to stop the buzzing and the spinning that's taking over my brain. How long is this going to last? I wish it would stop for just a second.

I open my eyes and Vickie is there in the front with all the other people standing close, all giving me worried looks. Their faces are so different, different shapes, different noses, different mouths that all seem to be moving. They won't forget this.

I see the child that had his hands on me. He reminds me of my Sammy, looks like he's about four, the same age that Sammy was when he died. He has blonde hair and green eyes, just like Sammy. He moves closer to me, and I can see that it is Sammy.

It is Sammy.

His grandmother is walking towards me now, but I know that it's not his grandmother; it's mine. They never met each other. How is this? They stand, smiling at me, quiet in the middle of all the other noise. I blink to make them go away, to focus so I can see who they really are.

They don't change.

They're the same as the days they both died, nine and a half years apart.

I'm crying and I feel like I may throw up. There is a hot-water rush under my tongue. I swallow hard to push the well back down.

They're standing right here, two feet in front of me. They've moved in front of Vickie now. They're calm, both of them.

My grandmother is wearing a pair of black moccasins I made for her when I was about fourteen, not long before she died. She sees me looking at her feet, and she wiggles her toes in them, picking at me.

Sammy's got on his shoes that light up in the heel when he walks. Good, he won't fall in here with those shoes on.

I want to touch them, and I reach out with both hands.

"Tambri, honey, don't do that," Vickie says and she catches my arms, stopping me from falling out of the chair.

"Here come the guys with the stretcher, okay?" Vickie says.

I look into Vickie's eyes, and I want to tell her who is here.

"Okay," is all I say. I look back for them; they're gone. The tears flow constant, making the pain throb. I close my eyes as they lift me on the gurney.

"Tambri, let go," Vickie says.

I feel her unwrap my fingers from a box I'm holding.

It's a DVD. Funny.

ↄ

Her nametag says *Alice,* and she watches me from time to time while I stare at her hair. It's crazy curly brown hair with gray in it. She's short and squatty and I feel the weight of her hands on my arm as she takes my blood pressure. She seems nice, smiling at me. I think maybe Alice is in her late fifties. I'm trying to focus on her eyes, but her hair is too distracting, and there is so much hair, it's hard for me to focus on one strand.

"You're going to be just fine," she says and pats my knee.

I feel like a kid lost in the mall. Everything is big and out of shape. My head throbs with a heavy thump inside my brain, and then another, like it's trying to remind me of something.

The way I've been feeling for so many years came out with the swing to the head. "Play ball," I say. Swing at will. An oncoming car, the morning alarm, a tornado, a nail sticking up from a two by four, the death of a child, a baseball bat.

Things you don't see coming.

A nurse is taking x-rays of my brain. She shifts my head in a different direction each time, leaves me and steps behind a wall, pushes something that makes a loud beep, comes back, shifts my head again, and goes back behind the wall. It isn't Alice; this girl is young and not friendly at all. Did she have a fight with her boyfriend, or is it that she doesn't like people, or is it that she doesn't like me, or she doesn't like her job, or she doesn't like going behind the wall every few minutes, or maybe she has a sad kind of face, or she's tired and doesn't want to carry on a conversation with someone who has a concussion from the looks of the X-rays.

I can't remember her name. I looked at her tag when she came in, but I can't see the letters in my head, and she's moving too fast now for me to read it. Maybe Alice's name isn't Alice.

"We're done," the girl says. She props the door open and wheels me out on the gurney. She hands me back over to Alice who's waiting in the hallway.

"I'll take her to her room," she says, over my head, talking to the girl.

Benny had to make Vickie leave. They stood by my bed in the emergency room before I was taken back. She wanted to stay with me, but he told her no. There was no reason for her to stay. She needed to let the "folks" at the hospital do their jobs. I don't know if I've ever heard him say "folks" before.

Vickie kissed the air above my head, not wanting to hurt me, and then walked to the door, waiting for Benny.

"You will be okay, Tambri," Benny said, almost commanding it to happen. Then he took my hand and kissed it like a gentleman, or a knight. It made me want to cry again, but I didn't because I knew it would make my head hurt more.

Alice is pulling me into my room. The wheels squeak as she makes a left with me. An orderly has followed us in, helping Alice to lift me onto the bed.

Alice takes my arm and a needle pricks my skin. I close my eyes and drift to sleep as she does her job around me.

I open my eyes and my room is dark except for one light behind my head. I hear the footsteps of a nurse coming down the hall. She's headed to my door. I can tell by the way she's walking. I can feel that she's coming for me.

She opens the door and there she is.

I search for her name. *Patti.*

I didn't realize how important it is to know someone's first name when you're laid up in a hospital. Maybe I'll get a name tag for my job. Most people are scared of seeing their own blood being taken.

I usually tell them my name, but I don't think they hear it sometimes.

Some of them just have a buzzing in their ears from the fear. It's not normal, they think. And it's not. Not an everyday thing anyway. I do need to get a *Tambri* nametag. I'll make sure to do that when I get back to work.

"Hey, Patti."

"Hey, Tambri," Patti says back to me, picking up my chart and walking towards my monitors.

"Are you feeling less dizzy?"

"Maybe a little." The bed seems to move just as she asks the question. She can tell things aren't right with me, with my head. She leans in checking my pupils like Vickie did. I'm guessing Patti knows more about pupils than Vickie does.

"We just need to watch you for a while. You'll be okay."

"I've never been that, Patti."

Patti laughs for my sake. I wonder if she's been talking with Alice or whatever her name is about my injury.

"Patti, I saw him today; my grandmother standing right beside him."

"Who?" she says and she writes something important about me on the chart.

"My son Sammy. My grandmother was standing right beside him."

"Where was this?"

"In the store, right after I got clocked in the head."

"Oh?"

"They're both dead, and they didn't say anything. God, I miss them, Patti. I miss them now, especially in this dark room."

"I know, Tambri," she says, and offers me some water by leaning the cup toward my face, holding the straw, so that I can reach it. I take a couple of sips.

"Thanks," I say.

"I'll see you in a couple of hours. Okay?"

"Okay."

I wait for Patti to come back as soon as she leaves. I think about her in my head trying to remember exactly what she looks like. She's a black lady in her late forties. She's a little heavy, but it doesn't look bad on her, and she's tall. I like her presence. She eased my mind a little, just her being in the room. Some people have that effect. The calmness rubs off. The energy of that person mixes with your energy and changes it.

I wish she was still here.

There's a clock to the right side of the blank T.V. I think the time is 2:40. At 4:40, Patti will be back. She said two hours. The face of the clock plays a game with me, shifting the hands just as I'm figuring it out. Does it say 1:30? I think I've got it, then I get confused and I'm not sure. This is draining.

From the very start it's been draining. Draining—like pulling a plug from a sink and the liquid spirals down. I'm the liquid in the drain, spinning down a dark metal tube that doesn't seem to stop. Dark metal tube. Maybe, that's why I've had so many husbands. No one wants to go down a dark metal tube by themselves. Bring someone with you who knows the feeling and it may not seem so scary. Or, maybe it's just as frightening, but you're just not alone. No, wait, that's just a tiny part of it. It's about me getting what I deserve.

What time is it?

I can hear footsteps again. I'm glad. I don't like being in here alone.

I can't seem to stop looking at the clock, struggling to figure out the time. I shut my eyes trying to avoid it.

Two people are coming in. Maybe it's a different shift, and Patti is telling the new person what she needs to know.

I open my eyes.

My grandmother and my son stand on opposite sides of my bed, peering at me. Sammy climbs onto the bottom rung of the bed so that we can see each other better. He leans forward on the metal rail, grinning at me.

It's too much for me to see them. I try to stop myself from crying, but I can't, and my head pounds with a steady pressure.

My grandmother slides her feet, moving her little body closer to me. She smells like she just took a bath, and the scent of her settles me. I wipe my face with the top of my sheet, and breath deep. I close my eyes and count each time I inhale.

I open my eyes wide and look at Sammy.

He laughs, and looks at my grandmother, as if he's telling me to look her way, too. I study Sammy for one second more, taking in his every line. I turn my head, and my grandmother watches me, smiling.

"Enough of this, honey, enough," she says softly, and the sound of her voice comforts me. She puts her fingers to her lips and blows me a kiss.

I close my eyes, and the warmth of them touches me. There is a melting in my stomach, and I feel something lift out of me. I can't put a name to it. I feel light and the lightness almost makes me laugh. Like the girl who took the X-Rays, I'll never know the name for this.

Rings

Every ring runs through me. The phones echo in offices down the hall, and it sounds like they say, "Your wife is not the same. Your wife is not the same." I struggle to focus on my job; I make calls. "Hello, I'm Eric Wilson," I say, smiling on my end so it comes across over the phone, while I work at cajoling people into buying life insurance, something they don't want or don't want to think about. And while I'm smiling and selling, the thought pricks at my brain, "Your wife is not the same."

Last night was different. The four of us were in the living room, like we usually are. Ella fell asleep in my arms while I was rocking her on the couch.

"Do you want to take her up to bed?" I said to Audrey. Almost always, I'm the one to put Ella to bed, but I thought maybe Audrey might enjoy saying goodnight to her daughter.

"No, you can do it," she said, popping the pages of a *People* magazine, glancing at the pictures.

That's not the first time I've asked her and she's said no. It's happening more and more. I guess last night wasn't that out of place from any other time with Audrey. She seems indifferent about everything, but sometimes it's more than that, she seems annoyed.

How can a mother not want to take her child to bed? This is the thing that scares me. She's done things before that make it not so easy for me to trust her, but she's never been this way with the kids.

She turned a picture of Reese Witherspoon toward me and said, "Do you think I can be as skinny as her in three weeks?"

"What happens in three weeks?"

"Nothing, I'm just giving myself a time limit to get this baby fat off of me," she says, pinching the top of her thigh through her jeans.

"You look good to me," I said. She's been talking about getting the baby weight off ever since Ella was born. Sometimes I wonder if she resents the baby for the extra pounds.

"That doesn't really count. You're married to me. What do other people think when they see my fat ass walking through the door at Chick-fil-a?"

"I don't know, Audrey. That you're hungry, and you're there to get something to eat?"

I couldn't figure out what the hell it was she wanted me to say. I'm not sure if she wants me to say anything at all. The way she looks at me sometimes makes me feel like a coat rack or something.

Everett laughed when Audrey cussed. He's nine, so cuss words are hilarious. Cuss words and farts. Of course, farts are one way that fathers and sons bond, so I laugh at the farts, too. He didn't miss a beat playing his "Warriors" game, splattering a black tank against a brick wall.

She looked toward Everett like she just realized he was in the room. "Everett, it's time to go to bed," she said.

"Mom, I've got thirty-eight more minutes," he said looking straight ahead to his game.

"Well, you're going to have to stop playing that game. It's giving me a headache."

Everett reached over to the remote on the floor beside him and turned the sound down.

"Damn good compromise," I said trying to make Everett laugh. It worked. He fell backwards on the floor laughing and sat right back up, still laughing and playing the game.

Audrey stood up, looked at me like she wanted me to say something to Everett. When I didn't, she stomped out of the room, making sure to leave her finger in the magazine where she had left off.

I asked Ed Robinson about it this morning. He works in the same department as me. He and his wife have four kids. I thought it might be the post-partum thing. Sandy went through it with their first child, Caleb. They gave all their kids names from the Bible. I think Ed is a deacon at his church.

Audrey came up with our kids' names. Before we had Everett, she said she wanted our children's names to start with the same letter as mine. "What about A for you?" I said laying my head on her still flat stomach. "No, I want them to be like you," she said.

I would have argued with her about it, but I thought I would get my way with our second child. I'd always heard to never disagree with a pregnant woman. Then she came up with the name Ella, and it seemed like a perfect name, and I didn't want to make a thing out of it. I wonder why she wanted to keep herself separate. It's something that nags at me once in a while, and then I forget about it. With the way she's acting, I'm glad the kids don't have A's for the first letter of their names.

Ed asked me if Audrey was crying all the time.

"No," I said.

Then he asked me if she was sleeping a lot.

"No," I said.

"Sandy was crying and sleeping all the time. I was worried. I wouldn't let her have the keys to the car. If she wanted to go somewhere, I took her."

He shook his head and said it didn't sound like what Sandy had. "What is she doing?" he said.

"Acting different, weird." I couldn't bring myself to tell Ed that Audrey doesn't seem to want to be a part of our children's lives. I didn't want to make her out to be a bad mother.

"I don't think that's what it is," he said. He shook his head some more and walked out of my office.

I don't think that's what it is either.

Audrey's always been the kind of person to compare herself and her life to everyone else. Does she have enough? Is she doing the right thing? She tries to find out what's going on in other people's homes, what car is in their garage, who is sleeping in their beds.

She used to talk about this girl at work that was the same age as her and hadn't gotten married. Actually, she might have been a couple of years older than Audrey.

"Don't you think it's funny that she's never gotten married?" she asked me one morning while I ate a piece of dry toast. We had run out of butter the day before.

"No, some people don't ever get married," I said between bites.

"I just think it's weird. She's had boyfriends and everything, so I know she likes men."

"I don't know, Audrey."

"She says it's because of her career, but I find that hard to believe. Don't you think most women still want to get married more than they want to have a career?"

I can't believe it when she says stuff like that. I don't think I know any other woman who would say that. I can't figure out if it's a good thing or a bad thing.

"No, some women don't."

"That just bothers me. It's not normal."

I shook my head at that.

"What, you think it is?"

"I didn't say that."

"Maybe I can fix her up with someone from your office."

This went on for about five more minutes, and I wanted her to stop hounding the poor girl who wasn't there to defend herself or the way she's decided to live her life.

Finally, I had to say, "I'll see if there's someone at the office that knows a single guy to set her up with. Okay?"

"Yes, that is perfect," she said and she acted like it made her feel a lot better. I'm not sure why it bothered her in the first place.

℘

Audrey is a good person. She can't stand to see someone get hurt; it's almost like she feels it herself. I broke my wrist moving furniture in the house. This was before the kids. I was trying to lift one side of the armoire to put it on top of a blanket, so that I wouldn't scratch the floor when I moved it from one side of the room to the other. I lost my hold on it and one leg fell on my right wrist. It was all I could do to lift up the armoire and off of my hand.

"I told you not to try to move that by yourself," Audrey said to me, and I could see her eyes watering. She'd been out with her friend Gail shopping.

"I'm okay; the doctor said it would be okay. It's just going to take time."

"Honey, I'm sorry," she said and lightly touched the splint. "Why didn't you call me? I should have gone with you."

"I didn't think it was broken. It didn't hurt that bad. I could drive."

"Does it hurt now?"

"Just a little, not too much. They gave me a prescription for pain if I need it."

"I'm going to get that for you. First, I need to set you up on the couch."

And she did. She tucked a clean sheet over the couch and brought me a pillow with a fresh pillowcase on it. She helped me put my pajama bottoms and T-shirt on, both out of the clean clothes basket.

"We need to keep everything clean."

"Audrey, it didn't break the skin," I said.

"Now, just relax. Here's the remote for the T.V., only use your left hand." She kissed me on the head and left with my prescription tucked inside the same hand holding onto the strap of her purse.

She was that way the entire time I healed. She'd help me wrap my cast in a plastic bag with a rubber band to close the opening around the top. Every morning, before I took my shower, she did this. She was constant and steady.

And every time I kissed her, it was deep, and warm, and I didn't want to let go.

When Dr. Sorenson said I had healed just like I should have, I almost wished that Audrey wasn't sitting in the chair beside me.

She was distracted as we walked to the car.

"It's good news, Audrey. The first time I came here, he told me that sometimes that bone doesn't heal like it's supposed to. Cartilage fills the gap instead of bone."

"What, why didn't you tell me?" She was concerned again.

"I guess I thought you were worrying enough."

We both climbed in the car, and I turned the key.

"That's my job." She rubbed my hand on the steering wheel.

"I'm glad it's all better," she said, and then she was gazing out the window.

"I need to let everybody know how good a healer my husband is," she said smiling as she pulled her phone out of her purse to call everyone to give them the good news.

"Gail, he's all better. And you know what, it might not have healed."

"I know. He didn't want to bother me with worrying about it."

She'd found a little something to fill her time.

❧

Ella's fast asleep in her room. I checked on her about twenty minutes ago. It's Saturday, so Everett didn't have school. He spent the night at his friend Dustin's house. It was Dustin's birthday, and he had a sleepover for about four of his friends. I wouldn't have wanted to be the parents in that house last night.

"How do I look?" Audrey says standing in front of me with jeans and a tight blue T-shirt and no shoes.

"You look good. You always do," I say smiling, reaching for her from the end of the bed. She swings her rear end away from me. She'd called me in here to show me something. I'd been waiting five minutes for her while she was in the bathroom. I didn't know what she was doing.

"Can't you tell?" she says. She angles her arms away from her body, keeping them straight and bends her wrists so that her hands point outward. She wants me to look at her body, and I have no problem with that.

"Are those new jeans?" I say laughing. I know what she wants me to say, but she wants me to say it so badly.

"Damn it, Eric," she says putting her hands on her waist.

"I'm just messing with you. You've lost weight. How much?"

"You can tell?" she says in a much brighter voice.

I nod my head.

"I haven't weighed myself in the last three weeks. That was the deadline I gave myself. I just wanted to get in these jeans, and look!" She turns in slow motion, smiling in the mirror, stepping on tiptoes to look at how small one side of her butt has gotten.

"Would you like some help out of those jeans, Mrs. Wilson?" I reach for her again, and I catch her by the arm and pull her toward me.

"Stop, Eric, that's not why I asked you to come in here. I just wanted to see if you could tell."

"Yeah, and now I want to get a closer look." I kiss her on the neck, and she goes limp.

"What?" I say.

"That's not what I want," she says and slides out of my hold. She grabs her silver sandals, and leaves me alone in our bedroom.

"Fine," I say under my breath.

"I'm going off with Gail. I'll be back in a couple of hours," she yells as she walks down the stairs. I can hear the tap of her shoes on the tile floor as she opens the door, walks out, and shuts it behind her.

It's quiet here. I lay back on the bed with my legs still off the end, and look at the light above my head. It's flickering a little. Is that the bulb or do I need to change out the wiring on that? I close my eyes.

I think distrustful things sometimes. Especially, when she leaves the house without me or without one of the kids with her, or, when Gail doesn't pick her up. It's all about her leaving alone.

When Everett was six and had just started first grade, Audrey started acting different.

She wasn't leaving the house by herself or anything. She just acted distant. I thought maybe something was wrong with her physically.

"Are you okay?" I said several times.

"I'm fine, Eric," she would say and laugh. "Why do you keep asking me that?"

"I don't know. I'm just concerned."

"Oh, honey, that is sweet, but I promise you that there is nothing wrong with me."

She didn't want me to touch her, I could tell that. She'd pretend to be asleep or tired. It didn't matter what time of day it was.

She didn't really want to talk about how her day went or ask me about mine.

She would stay up late on the computer. She said she was talking to Gail. Apparently, Gail was having a hard time with her divorce. I could understand why Audrey wanted to try to help her, but it was almost every night.

"Why is it you aren't too tired for her, but you are too tired for me?" I would say.

"This is different. We aren't doing anything physical," she would say.

"Why do you have to talk to her so late?" I said.

"That's usually when she gets lonely and starts thinking about things."

"What do you talk about for that long?"

"We talk about what a jerk Ronnie is and how he doesn't deserve her."

"For three hours?"

"Well, sometimes we play games over the internet. You know—just something to pass the time."

"Honey, how long is this going to go on? You need your sleep and I do, too."

"Not much longer, but I'm not sure. I can't leave her hanging out there."

"Doesn't she have a sister? Can't you and her sister take turns talking to her so late at night? You wake up in the morning with blue circles under your eyes. You have to think about yourself, too."

"I will. I promise," and she'd kiss me on the mouth and turn around to the computer.

About 2:00 o'clock one morning, I woke up and Audrey still wasn't in bed. This is enough, I thought.

I decided that I was going to let Gail know that this was just too much. She was pushing the limits of Audrey's friendship.

I walked in my socks to the bedroom that we use as an office. Thinking back now, I didn't make any noise as I walked through the door.

Audrey was laughing at something on the screen. I guessed that Gail was feeling better. I thought this was a good time to break up the conversation and get my wife in bed where she should be.

She was still laughing when I walked up behind her, and I guess she didn't hear me. She started typing, and I read the line that was there before, from jimmyc123@ something. I didn't read the rest of the address, just what was written.

My feet are shaped like penguins. I wish you could see them; I got these from my great-aunt Mimi. Of all things to get from her, I wish I'd gotten her thick mustache.

What the hell is this? I thought.

I held my breath as Audrey finished typing.

From the picture I saw, I don't think you need a mustache anyway. You're handsome without it.

"What the hell is this?" I said to Audrey's back, and I said it loud enough to wake Everett, but I didn't know it at the time.

She turned around and stared up at me. I wanted to slap her in the face. I knew exactly what this was.

"Oh, I'm just talking with my friend, Jimmy," she said.

"Where did Gail go?"

"Well, she was tired and had to go to bed."

"You weren't tired?" I said.

"No, I think I was so awake worrying about Gail."

"Who is Jimmy?"

"He's just somebody I met online."

"Online? Online where?"

"You know, just online. You know, I talk to different people online. We talk about what bugs us, and what we want to do with our lives," she said.

"What do you want to do with yours, Audrey?"

"Nothing, I was just talking, that's all, Eric," and then she had the dumbass idea to act insulted. "Eric, are you saying you don't trust me?"

I stared down at her. I couldn't believe what she was saying. She was trying to make me the bad guy. I looked at the screen again, and I could see Jimmy the jackass typing over and over again, *Are you there, Audrey?*

She could feel it, and she turned around to answer him. I wanted to pull her chair out from under her.

"What's going on?" I heard Everett say from behind me.

"Nothing, Everett," Audrey said as she hit return on the computer to send her last message. She shut it down with the button so it would turn off in a hurry, and I couldn't see what she had written.

She got up and didn't look at me. She took Everett's hand and said, "Come on, sweetheart, I'll put you back in bed." Then she left me standing there.

I stood there going through what I'd seen and what she had said to me. Was I being a jealous husband? And then I remembered the way she looked when she turned around and realized I was standing behind her.

Her mouth opened just a little like she was in shock. She didn't move her head up to look at me; she only moved her eyes.

I pulled the computer plug out of the wall and every other plug I could find connected to something. I picked up the monitor, and I thought about throwing it out of the window from the second floor, but I knew that would give Audrey something to hang on to. "I can't believe you made such a big deal out of nothing. And then you decide to throw the computer out the window. How am I supposed go walking down our street, again? You embarrassed the hell out of me in our own neighborhood," she would have said.

So, I carried everything out to the car, drove it to the dumpster at Burton's Bar on Francis Street, and tossed it in. I meant that she wasn't going to use it again.

Audrey tried to talk to me about jimmyc123 a couple of times.

"Nothing happened," she would say. That's the way she'd always try to start the conversation. I walked out of whatever room we were standing in. She never tried to talk about it in the car; I guess she was afraid of what I might do.

❧

"What?" I say, still flipping the channels because there isn't a damn thing on. I'm really only going back and forth between a show about fixing up old cars and seeing how much their worth, and a documentary about the Vietnam War.

My mom's in town from Virginia, and she's out with the kids spoiling them some more.

Audrey's been mumbling something from the kitchen, and I've yet to hear what it is. I turn the sound down.

"What?"

"I'm moving," Audrey says.

"What?" I lean forward on the couch still watching the T.V.

"I'm moving." I thought that's what she said, but that doesn't make any sense.

"What do you mean?"

"Exactly what I said." Her voice lowers each time she says it. I strain harder each time to hear it. I leave the T.V. on and drop the remote on the couch as I stand up and walk into the kitchen. The kitchen's cleaner than I've seen it in a long time. The counters shine. I heard her working in here earlier. The brightness of the chrome on the refrigerator makes me uneasy. I walk over and look inside. It's spotless; everything that was old or sticky has been thrown out. Everything else is organized and clean. I close the door and turn toward Audrey.

She's sitting at the counter peeling an orange. There is a blue bowl containing some of the rinds.

"What does that mean?" I say, unable to stop myself from giving a nervous laugh.

"I'm moving to Panama City."

My skin tingles, charged from what she's just said.

"The kids are still in school. You've never even mentioned wanting to go to Panama City."

She continues with the orange. She's unpeeled the whole thing, and now she's pulling the slices apart. She focuses on the task. I realize she's not eating it; she drops each piece into the bowl, her hands covered in juice.

"This is something that we need to discuss," I say. "I didn't think you liked Florida that much. Remember, I asked you if you wanted to go there last summer." My breath is coming faster, and the words feel like drying cement in my mouth.

"I was seven months pregnant with Ella. Do you think that's the best time for a woman to go to Florida?"

She's trying to pick a fight. I know her; I've seen this before.

"You're right," I say. I sit down, across the counter from her.

"I'm moving to Panama City by myself."

I stare at her and lace my fingers together on top of the hard surface. It's cold under my palms, and my knuckles bow as I tighten my fingers.

"Do you plan on taking the kids with you?" It's hard enough to understand that she's leaving me. She keeps using the word I'm, not me and the kids. It's a terrible thing to swallow that she wants to leave me, but her children? That makes her a horrible, horrible person. It's miserable to think that I chose this person for my wife and the mother of my children.

"No, I'm not taking the kids."

"Son-of-a-Bitch, Audrey. What are you doing?"

"I need to try something different."

"Something different? You're talking about leaving your family—me, and Everett, and Ella. Ella who happens to only be seven months old." I'm yelling now, if there's any time to yell, it's now.

She's lost her mind.

"I don't know how long I'll be gone. It may not be forever."

"What, you think there's a way back in? If you leave and go to Florida, you won't be coming back in this house. Do you understand, Audrey?"

She pushes the bowl away from her and stands up. She turns to the sink and rinses her hands, her back to me.

"I thought with your mother being here and all that this would be the best time for me to leave. She can help you with the kids."

"Jesus, she's only here for three more days." Why am I talking about how long my mother will be here?

"Are you really going by yourself?" I say holding my breath as she walks out of the kitchen. I follow her as she heads up the stairs and into our bedroom.

"Answer me!"

She ignores me and picks up her suitcases that she must have packed when I wasn't in the house. There are three of them. I open our bedroom window. I snatch the two bags that are in her hands, and I throw them through the opening, busting the screen. I don't give a damn what the neighbors might think, and it's obvious that Audrey doesn't either.

"Now, you won't try to come back—will you? You'll be too embarrassed to be seen on this street. But you're sure as hell not too embarrassed to leave your family for some bastard. I wonder what the neighbors will think of that."

I know she has somebody else; she's not the kind of person to be by herself.

"What is his name?"

She picks up her last bag and starts walking away from me.

"What is his name, Audrey?"

She turns around and looks at me like she's about to stab me.

"Jim," she says.

I sit back on the edge of the bed, almost missing what Audrey said. She watches as the name sinks in more and more.

ᘒ

"Ella is your child," my mother says to me as I stand outside my car. Everett had school and Ella's taking a nap, after waking up at 3:30 this morning. I told Everett his mom went out of town to see a friend of hers.

"I have to make sure," I tell my mom. It's been three days since Audrey left, and it hit me the first night. How long has she been seeing him? Has it been ever since I threw the computer in the dumpster at Burton's? If she's been seeing him for that long, how do I know that Ella is mine?

"You don't have to."

"How do you know?"

My fifty-seven-year-old mother stands in front of me with her uncombed gray and blonde hair while her arms burn in the sun. "Because if she belonged to that asshole Audrey left with, Audrey would have taken Ella with her."

"Mom, I don't think she gave a damn who Ella belonged to. No matter what, Ella's her child, and she left her."

"You've got to think more about what you're about to do."

"I don't want to think about this. I just want to know something for sure."

"Besides, don't you love that child that's in there sleeping like nothing's wrong. Do you want her to find out about this someday, because somebody in the doctor's office runs their big mouth?"

"Mom, my appointment's at 10:30." I get in the car, close the door, make sure she backs up from the car, and drive off not looking at her.

I'm not going to the doctor. My mother's right; I can't do that to Ella. I just couldn't stand there listening to my mother anymore. I didn't want to talk about it anymore.

I'm driving, and everything, and I mean everything, is running through my head. How long has she been seeing this guy? How long has she been planning to leave with him? How long, how long, how long?

I think about every small thing she's done that seems weird. This is what the weight was about, and the looking in the magazines and not taking care of her child. I wondered if there was someone else, but I didn't think it was the same bastard from before. She asked me how she looked before she went off to see him. God, that's messed up.

Her friend Gail hasn't called the house since this has happened. I keep hoping she will, so that I can see if she'll say anything about all of this. It's strange that she hasn't called. In the evenings, she calls the phone in the house because Audrey usually leaves her cell phone in her purse. Gail knows

Audrey can get to one of the phones in the house quicker than she can the phone in her purse.

Gail knows what has happened; that's why she hasn't called. Damn it, how long has she known about this? Did she know that Audrey was leaving?

Maybe she helped talk Audrey into this? This all started, as far as I know, when Gail was getting her divorce. Maybe it made Audrey think about other things? Maybe Gail is partly to blame for this.

I turn the car around and head toward Shepherd Avenue; Gail works there. She's the receptionist at a dentist office, mine and Audrey's dentist. He used to be Audrey's dentist. That's how Gail and Audrey became good friends. Audrey would stand at the little window talking to Gail about each other's kids and being mothers, and what things kids did that were similar, and what drove them crazy.

I pull into the parking lot, and Gail is standing at the side of the building smoking a cigarette. Strange that someone who works for a dentist smokes. She stands with her shoulders slumped like she always does, and she looks up. She sees me. She drops the cigarette, smashes it under her foot, and waits for me.

I'm stepping out of the car, and I can hear her say, "I didn't have a damn clue she was going to do this, Eric." She said my name in a sad way, her voice lower, like she felt sorry for me. I believe her.

I walk to the front of my car and sit on the warm hood. Gail moves closer to me by one step and the smoke smell comes with her.

"This is craziness," she says.

I nod my head.

"Why would she leave the kids?" she says. "Why would she leave you?"

I scrunch my shoulders up to say "I don't know." I'm afraid to talk. I'm afraid I'll break down right here at the dentist office, in front of Gail. This is ridiculous.

I swallow hard, trying to push down the welling sensation I feel in my chest. The last time I experienced something like this was when my father died. He died, for God's sake. Audrey's not dead. My breath is coming faster. I know Gail can see.

She takes two more steps and puts her hand on my shoulder.

"Do you want me to help you find a daycare for Ella?" she says, looking me straight in the eye like she doesn't know I'm on the verge of falling apart.

I haven't even thought about what I'm going to do with Ella during the day. Yes, I need a daycare. My breath slows down.

"Yes," I say, "I would appreciate that, especially since I don't know a damned thing about daycare," and I laugh.

She laughs, too. "Well, with three boys, I know a lot." She squeezes my shoulder and lets go.

☙

Audrey's the reason why I started working at Sherman's Insurance. I've been there ten years now. It's boring as hell, but if you work hard enough, you can make some money. I wanted to keep her happy. Sometimes that wasn't the easiest thing to do when I could feel her always looking over my shoulder, checking to see if there was something better behind me.

I'm going to put my notice in today with Mr. Sherman. He's always treated me well; I think he deserves a notice, even with everything that's going on with me.

"Good luck to you," he says while he shakes my hand hard and looks me straight in the eye.

"Thank you, sir." Mr. Sherman's always had a military feel to him: shoulders back, head up, chest out. I've always felt the need to call him sir.

It's been good of Mom to leave her second husband, Dan, up in Virginia by himself for so long. He's a good guy; he's good to my mom. He owns a sporting goods store up there. He told her to stay down here as long as I need the help. She was only supposed to be here a week.

"You know I can stay for two more weeks," she told me as soon as Audrey pulled her leaving town act. "I would stay longer, but I don't have any more time at work." She works for a grocery store. She's over the deli department.

I wanted to tell my mother no, she didn't have to stay at all, but what else could I do? I don't have anyone else to take Everett to school, and I certainly don't have anyone around here I trust enough to keep Ella all day. The daycare that Gail helped me find isn't able to get Ella in for about a month. Audrey had decided she wouldn't go back to work after Ella was born. We talked about it, and she said she wanted to stay home with her. I told her I could sell more to make up the difference.

That's a hell of a note; it makes me think that Audrey lied to me the whole time. It's hard to tell where the truth ended with Audrey. I don't know now if there ever was any truth to her.

I'm going to start doing electrical work again, after my two-week notice is up. That is, if I can beg the people at Friendly Fran's Daycare to take Ella sooner. If there really is a Fran, I'm going straight to her.

"I can work around the kid's schedule if I'm working for myself," I told my mom while we both stood in my kitchen a couple of nights ago. Both the kids were in bed. I told Everett his mom would be out of town for a few more days. I'll tell him the truth when I get used to it a little more.

"Good, you always enjoyed working with your daddy," she said while she was wiping off the counters in the kitchen.

"Yeah, he was good at what he did," I said.

"Made a pretty good living at it. We never went hungry," she said laughing, making the lines around her eyes deeper.

My mom hadn't mentioned Audrey since our conversation outside of my car.

"What do you do to get over something like this?" I said while I looked in the refrigerator for something that might appeal to me. Every time I look in that spic and span refrigerator, I can almost feel my blood pressure go up. I slammed the door.

"I know you've heard this before, but you've got to give it time," my mom said.

"How much?"

"All depends on the person."

"Do you think Audrey will come back?"

"I hope not. She'll just do more damage," she said and left me in the kitchen with my coffee. Audrey is gone, gone, gone, as far as my mother is concerned.

❧

My first couple of electrical jobs take me about three times as long as they should have. I'm used to my dad being there, and sometimes it takes a while to think on your own when you're used to somebody else kind of directing you.

Plus, I haven't done work like this in over ten years. I've done things around the house like changing the switch in the living room from a regular switch to a dimmer switch. I've kept up my license because Dad made me promise that I would.

"It's a good trade, a really good trade," he would say. I believed that it was a good trade, but I never thought after I married Audrey that I would be doing this kind of work again. You can make a good living at it, but the work is never steady. And that's where Audrey wouldn't have put up with me doing this kind of work. She always wanted a steady income coming in. Always.

And then she left, and I needed flexibility. Audrey was never flexible, unless I count her leaving her family. That is pretty damn flexible about things.

Today is Ella's birthday. She turned one. It's a big number. Did Audrey call or email to ask for a picture? Did she send anything?

Of course, if she had sent anything, I would have thrown it away.

❧

"Everett, you are getting so good at this game," I say to my son and I throw the baseball back to him. I can feel the heat of the ball when he throws it to me. He gets better and better each time we practice.

He played T-ball for a couple of years when he was little, maybe four or five. He asked me last summer, after his mom left, if he could start playing again. I told him I thought it was a good idea. It's an easy game for him, not that he doesn't work hard at it. He does. He plays a couple of positions, sometimes pitcher, sometimes shortstop. The season starts in about two weeks, and we've been out here most evenings practicing.

Ella plays in her sand box while we practice. Me and Everett built it for her, and all three of us went to the store to get the sand. It took four big bags to fill it. We all sat in it that day and played in the dirt. Ella loves it.

I squat to be the catcher and give Everett the two-finger signal. He nods and burns the curve ball to me. I stand up and throw the ball back to Everett harder than I ever have to him. He's strong enough to take it. "That is how you throw a curve ball," I tell him pointing at him with my gloved hand.

"That was a good one?"

"Yep, the best one I've seen you throw."

He grins and winds up to throw again. I get into position.

"I wish Mom were here to see it," he says and releases the ball. There is no force behind the ball.

And with that, Audrey has punched Everett in the stomach, knocked the breath out of him, right in the middle of what was supposed to be a fastball.

I thought this would get his mind off of her. Concentrating on something physical, something where you have to focus. But there's always room for her to step up and present herself.

Everett hurts the most. He always will. Ella doesn't remember her, so she'll pretty much be okay. But Everett was old enough when she left to remember everything. I'm sure he even remembers how she smelled. I'm an adult, and I can find ways to deal with this. Plus, I still have my mother. Everett doesn't, and that pisses me off.

When Everett was about three, we all went to the Grand Canyon. I remember it was hot and windy. I stood there holding Everett so he wouldn't get too close to the metal railings, and Audrey stood beside us. We all looked at the massive hole before us.

I have images of that now, but Everett's not there. It's just me and Audrey standing by the edge, and there's no security barrier. She's not even facing the canyon; her body is turned to the side, and she's flipping the pages of a magazine while the hot wind moves her hair and skirt. She keeps showing me pictures of things she wants and how she wants to look like the women in the magazine.

And then, when she turns the magazine back to herself, and she's the most intrigued by the glossy pages, I reach over and push her by the shoulder.

❧

I'm working on a house; well really, I'm just hanging a light outside. The people, Gena and Walter Suddeth, were actually really good friends with my dad and mom, even though they were a good ten years older than my parents.

I've always liked both of them. Me and my father did the electrical work on their addition about fifteen, maybe sixteen years ago.

Gena called me at home last night, and asked me if I could put a light up at her house.

"Yep, I can definitely do that," I told her. It was good to hear her voice.

She and Walter have been standing here, talking to me the entire time I've been working. Not that I mind at all.

"You know why you're putting up that light, don't you, Eric?" Gena says looking up at me as I stand on the second to the top rung of the ladder leaning against the side of the house.

"Tell me, Gena." She already told me on the phone last night, but I know she wants to tell me again in front of Walter.

"Because Walter was out here, too late, after I told him not to be, picking up limbs and working on the yard, and he stepped in a hole and sprained his ankle."

"That's too bad, Gena," I said yelling down to her.

Walter just watches me work.

"He's stubborn, Eric."

"So I've heard," I say.

"Even though he's sprained his ankle, and I've told him not to be out here that late in the evening, he's going to do it again."

"You think so, Gena?" I'm laughing now.

"Yep, and that is the reason why you are putting the light up."

"Good to know," I say, and I climb down to the ground and face Gena and Walter smiling.

"You talk too much, Gena," Walter says.

"Walter, go inside and get the money that we owe, Eric."

Walter obeys and heads toward the side entrance of the house.

"You don't have to pay me now, Gena."

"Of course, I'm paying you now. This is how you make your living. You've got kids to feed."

"Yep, Everett does try to eat everything he can find in the kitchen."

"I'm sorry all this happened to you, Eric."

"Well, it's getting better," I say, looking down at the ground.

"I want to tell you something," she says, and I can tell it's important.

"Okay," I say, waiting.

"I know that the man that Audrey left town with broke up with her. Left her down there all by herself."

"I don't…" I can't think of anything else to say. My tongue feels numb.

"I know you didn't want to hear anything about her, but I just didn't want you to hear it from someone else that you didn't know."

I stare at Gena. She grabs my hand and squeezes it hard, bringing me out of my stupor.

"Thanks, Gena. I appreciate you telling me."

❧

The phone's ringing, and I'm standing outside on the steps with the kids. I push the door open with my knee and release both their hands.

"Everett, can you take your little sister to the bathroom, please?" She's been saying she's had to go for the last fifteen minutes in the car.

He takes his sister's hand and leads her.

"You can't come in the bathroom with me, Everett."

"I don't want to," he says.

"Daddy, make sure Everett doesn't come in the bathroom with me."

"He won't," I say, heading toward the ringing.

I know it's got to be Gena on the phone. She's called me two times to confirm that I'll come back next week to do some electrical work for them inside the house. Gena had asked when I had finished putting up the outside light if I could check out the electrical inside the house.

"I want to see if anything else needs to be done," she said pushing me into their garage and into the house.

Lots of things need to be done, and some of it may be a hazard. I don't want anything happening to them because of something that I could have fixed. I'm a little out of breath from getting the kids in the door and running to catch the phone.

I pick up the receiver.

"Hey, I had to run to the phone," I say. There is a pause, and I know that it isn't Gena on the other end. I sit on the arm of the couch.

"I called your work number," Audrey says.

Did you, now? I think, and my head is on fire.

"I'm not there anymore, Audrey," I say, and my mouth barely moves as the feel of her name chokes me. I cough, and I want to spit.

"I talked to Ed; he told me," she says. Her voice is calm. She's rehearsed this; she's purposely not getting upset. She's hoping she can ride this first conversation out.

"Yep, Ed's a pretty smart guy. He didn't think you had post-partum depression."

"No?" she says, still in the same monotone.

"No," I say yelling. I remember the kids, and I lower my voice. "Boy, was he right." I decided sarcasm can work just as well, maybe even better, than yelling. And the kids won't have to hear any of this.

There is a long pause. She's regrouping. I'm wondering what she's going to come up with next.

"How's Ella?"

I stand up from the couch.

"Bigger, much bigger. You wouldn't know her," I say, sitting on the *know* for as long as I can. "Her hair is even darker."

"You don't think I would know her?" she says.

"Audrey, she wouldn't know you."

"That's my fault, I guess." Her voice is changing, anger creeping in. What does she have to be angry about? That's okay, though, I'm the one who's picking the fight this time.

"Yes, it sure as hell is. Don't you think?"

"How much do I need to pay for this?" She is really loud. She caught me off guard with the phone call, but I'm the one in charge now.

"I can't think of a number high enough," I say.

"I want to come home, Eric." She's being forceful now, almost demanding that I let her back into this house, into the lives of our children.

"Why?"

"Because the kids need their mother, and you need a wife."
I can almost see her stomping her foot, holding the phone to
her ear, surprised at how this is going.

"I don't think so."

"Am I supposed to pay for this forever?"

"I don't know, Audrey. Why don't you ask your boyfriend?"

"I wouldn't have to move right back in. I could come by
the house a couple of times a week, so the kids could get used
to me again. You would get used to me again." She's pleading
now. It's annoying.

"It is too late for that."

"No, that can't be right."

"Both of us should move on," and I'm about to hang up,
pulling the receiver away from my face, and I hear her say,
"I could take the kids from you."

I bring the phone back so fast that I hit my temple with the
top of it. "Listen, you are not their mother. Do you understand
me? You don't know anything about them, and I know that
you are too much into Audrey to take them by yourself."

"But Eric, I don't like being by myself. I don't like thinking
for myself."

She's crying.

"You'll find somebody. There's a lot of fish out there." My
patience and voice are strained.

"You think so?" she says.

"Yes, Audrey, I have no doubt you'll find someone. So,
yes, I think so."

She's about to say something else. I hang up and stare at
the phone. I look up as Everett and Ella tromp up the hallway
and back to me.

Curtains

I've decided no more men, no more husbands to fill in the time and the void. Doesn't that sound ridiculous? No more husbands. It makes me choke to say it out loud. Four total. Not as many as Elizabeth Taylor, but still way too many.

My goal has been not to bring any more men to my house. It's too close and way too intimate. And now, the horses' farrier, Carl, whose been changing the horse's shoes now for years, wants to bring one right to my door.

"Can't you fix the light in Sammy's room?" I ask Carl as he stands holding the fresh cup of coffee I just poured for him. I stand on the other side of the fence to the stables, and hold the half-empty coffeepot in my hand. Carl drinks about three pots of coffee a day, no matter how hot or cold it is outside. And today it's around ninety-seven degrees. I'd had my shoes off while I was in the house and walked outside through the hot dirt and clay to where Carl stood working on Benji's shoes.

"Tambri, I don't know anything about electricity. All I know is how to change a bulb and you said you did that already, and I know, too, that you shouldn't mess with electricity if you don't know anything about it."

I'm okay with Carl. He's a little older than me; I think he'll be forty-seven his next birthday. He's happily married to a rather large woman named Susanna. He loves her, and he's also a little scared of her, a combination that most men don't want to let go of.

"The next time I come out to check on the horses, I'll bring Eric with me. He can take a look and tell you what's going on."

What kind of name is that for an electrician? I think. I go through the alphabet to find a name that sounds more like an electrician. I end at C with Carl. Carl sounds more like an electrician's name than Eric.

I better lighten up on Carl. He's beginning to talk to me like he does with Susanna. His tone is almost a plea, begging me to understand that the only option is for Eric to come out to the house and take a look.

"Okay," I say, and I smile at Carl to let him know everything's fine.

"Eric really is a good guy, Tambri."

"I know, Carl. I trust you." I laugh, hoping the conversation is over.

"He's had a bad run of luck, too."

I hate to be pitied. That *too* said it all. I want to say, "Don't include me in any group with Eric." But I'm not going to say that to Carl.

"His wife ran off with this guy she was messing around with from the internet."

"Oh?" I say. That's the best I can come up with.

Carl loads his equipment into the truck and keeps talking, not really looking at me.

"Yep, she left about one-and-a-half, maybe two years ago. Left him and their two kids."

"So what?" I want to yell, and kick the dirt. "He still has the kids, doesn't he?" None of this comes out of my mouth. I don't kick anything, either.

"Thanks," I say. "Be careful heading home," and I wave as he pulls out. He waves back.

I walk toward the house, retracing my backward steps in the orange dust. My feet burn from standing in the sun talking to Carl. The ground blisters like white coals and send shocks from the tender part of my feet to the top of my brain. I run to the house and landed flat-footed on the cool white kitchen floor.

This whole thing makes me uneasy. I don't like the thought of a stranger in Sammy's room. Even Daniel stopped going in there after Sammy died. None of my other husbands ever went in the room. Not that I saw anyway.

It wasn't supposed to be this way. I've been fleeced of the package that I bargained for: a child and a husband. I had them both. Then one died, and the other couldn't take it and had to leave. Then other husbands started rolling in.

I wish I could fix the damn light myself.

I've tried putting a lamp in Sammy's room, but the room still seems too dark. I've sat in the room with the hallway light on at night, but it throws weird shadows. So, for the past month I've been sitting in the room each evening with all the lights off in that part of the house.

I don't want Sammy's room to be dark anymore. The fixture needs to be repaired by somebody who knows what he's doing.

I'll sit on the floor and watch the dark shapes grow longer as the sun disappears outside. Then the room turns to black, and I'm fixed in place right in the middle of it. A couple of nights ago, I felt a scream building in my chest. I sat there thinking it wouldn't matter if I did or didn't scream; no one would come to smooth my hair and soothe my nerves. The thought made me want to scream more.

Before I went completely over the edge, I groped my way to the door. I caught my breath during the walk to the living room. My legs, arms, and the base of my body trembled, even my tongue sitting snuggly in my mouth shook. I grabbed one forearm hard with my hand straining to make it stop. I turned on the television for company, and watched a commercial advertising the old Johnny Carson show episodes. It got my attention just enough.

❧

Today's the day Carl's bringing Eric with him. I've already started a pot of coffee for them. I'm not sure if Eric drinks it or not. I'm making it for Carl anyway. With Carl drinking all that coffee, you'd think he would shake like a leaf. He's got some of the steadiest hands I've ever seen. Well, except for my grandmother. She could have kept up with Carl with the coffee drinking, and the steady handedness.

Carl pulls up in his truck. The gravel and dirt shift under the weight of that big thing. I can hear it through the walls, and I see him through the kitchen window.

Susanna hates that truck. You almost have to have a ladder to climb into the thing.

I spread my hands against the waist of my cotton shirt, pressing out wrinkles that aren't there. Carl is climbing out, and there, of course, is Eric climbing out, too.

I walk out of the house, and toward both of them pasting a smile on my face. My skin is like granite, and it's all I can do to act cheerful.

"Hey, guys," I say.

"Hey, Tambri," Carl says. "This is Eric."

"Nice to meet you, Eric," I say.

He is not a bad-looking guy, around my age, early forties, slender. Eric offers his hand, and I shake it. His hand is worn with calluses, and the feel makes me look closer as he releases his grip. Some of the skin is cracked. He sees me looking, and he knows what I'm thinking.

"Sorry about that," he says rubbing both hands together.

"Shows you work hard," I try to say in a light tone. My mouth feels dry, scratchy.

"Of course he works hard. I wouldn't bring a slacker to your house, Tambri," Carl says. "Want me to take a look at Benji?"

"Yeah," I say and walk towards the house knowing that Eric will follow.

"Carl, a fresh pot of coffee is in the house," I yell back. I end up yelling into Eric's face. He moves quicker than I thought.

He laughs.

"Sorry about shouting in your face," I say.

"Not a big deal at all."

I lead him into the house and back to Sammy's room. I step just inside the door to the right; he follows behind me looking around the room. "I've done that before," he says looking toward the curtains, and he laughs a little.

Yesterday, I felt the need to wash everything that was made of cloth in Sammy's room. It's been so long since any company has been in his room. I shrank the curtains about three-inches. I laughed when I saw how short they were, but it doesn't mean Eric can laugh now.

He turns toward me, sees my face then looks around the room again, slower this time. Taking everything in as he backs up just a little facing me. He's figured it out; Carl wasn't brave enough to tell him.

"This is where the problem is?" Eric says.

"Yep, the light doesn't work at all. I changed the bulb."

"No good, huh?"

"Nope."

"Well, I'll go get my ladder and take a look."

We walk back out of the room together, and I point to the attic in case he needs to know where it is.

"Good to know," he says and smiles at me. I search for pity in the lines of his face. Like I said, I hate that. I don't really see any.

"Do you need me anymore?" I ask him and stop in the kitchen.

"Not right now, I'll just take a quick look and let you know what I think it is." He pushes the screen door open and heads back out into the heat.

I pretend to clean the kitchen. I pull old stuff out of the fridge and start throwing things in the garbage. There's more than I thought. I drag the trash can in front of the open refrigerator door.

Eric's moving past me now with the ladder. "Where's the fuse box?"

"Right beside the door." I point with something wrapped in crumpled aluminum foil.

"Will you turn off the one to Sammy's room?"

"The panel's not marked," I say.

"Can you flip each breaker until I see which one is the right one?"

"Yep."

"When the light goes out, I'll yell to let you know."

I nod.

He goes to Sammy's room, and I open the metal panel.

"Ready?" I yell.

"Go ahead."

"First one," I say and flip the switch.

"Not it, try again."

"How about now?"

"Yep, that's the one. That was quick," he says yelling louder, and laughing a little. I don't laugh back. I shut the metal box hard, and the sound bounces through the house.

My first husband Daniel had the same issue when the microwave went out in the kitchen. The problem was we couldn't have the toaster on at the same time as the microwave.

I'd turn on different appliances at different times to see what would flip the breaker.

I tried the stove and the toaster. That worked. I tried the stove and microwave. That worked. Sammy was watching from his high chair as I turned on different things while his daddy waited by the fuse box.

Then I tried the toaster with the microwave and the stove, toaster, refrigerator, and microwave turned off. We could hear the breaker flip.

Sammy clapped like it was some kind of magic trick. Daniel and I laughed with him.

"That's it, Tambri. We can't run the toaster and the microwave at the same time."

"Okay, then the toast will be the final course of this fabulous meal," I said, and kissed Daniel on the mouth holding my big plastic spoon in my hand. I reached down, and kissed Sammy on the head. I had taken him outside earlier, and his hair was matted with mud from playing. He smelled like he was part of the earth, just like little boys do.

I finished making breakfast and that was the end of that problem. Easy.

It sounds like Eric is in the attic now, and he is cussing like nobody's business. I can't help but laugh. I just didn't expect him to do that. Of course, how long have I known him, ten minutes?

Here he comes down from the attic, walking toward me into the kitchen.

"Tambri, this is a bigger problem than I thought."

I flinch a little when he uses my name. Why shouldn't he use my first name? That's how Carl introduced me to him.

"I'm guessing the house was built about mid-fifties."

"Fifty-four." I know because Daniel showed me the date under the lid of the toilet.

"I need to really get up there for a while, but just looking at the way things are at first glance, it looks like a lot of the house needs to be rewired."

No.

"I'll give you a fair price. If you want, I can just repair the problem in your son's room, but it really is dangerous to leave things the way they are."

I can't even talk. He's going to be around more than just today.

"If you want to think about it, Tambri, you definitely can."

Him saying my name again shakes me out of my dazed state.

"No, let's do it. Take a better look. Let me know how much. It has to be done." I laugh a little not wanting him to think I'm a nut.

"Yeah, it does."

"I mean I want to be able to sleep at night without worrying about it."

"I'd be worried, too."

೮೨

Eric's been back three times since the first visit. I'm kind of getting used to him coming by, working in the house. It's not so bad. It's nice to have somebody in the house doing something that doesn't need my attention. I like to hear noise in the house, noise that's not being made by me.

I hear his SUV outside. He said he was coming by. I made sandwiches for both of us. I'm guessing he may want to eat before he starts working.

Eric is talking to another person as the car doors open and close. It sounds like Eric's brought another man with him. Maybe he needs extra help today with what he's going to be doing. I listen as I set the cups on the table next to the sandwiches. I don't recognize the other voice, but I can hear that it's deep. There is a cracking sound that comes and goes in the man's voice.

I know who it is. It's Eric's son. He's brought his son to my house.

Eric told me that Everett's voice was changing. I sit down at the table, trying to listen to them talking as they walk closer to the door. Then I hear the girl's little voice, "Whose house is this, Daddy?"

I jump. A child that small hasn't been in this house since Sammy died. I catch my breath, reaching for the underside of the chair with both hands, holding on. Should I hide in the closet? I have hidden in a closet before. I was trying to avoid a boy who stopped by my grandma's house to see me.

What am I thinking? My car's outside, the lights are on, and they can probably see me through the window on the door. Plus, and I'm glad this has finally hit me, that I'm a grown woman, and I can't avoid letting them in.

But I'm scared of meeting those kids.

Eric has knocked twice now.

I bolt from the chair and stop myself from rushing to the door. I make myself slow down.

I open the door, and there they were. They all stop talking. The girl stands behind Eric's leg, peeking around the side. The boy drops his eyes and glances at me sideways.

"Hey," Eric says.

"Hey," I say just standing here.

"I hope you don't mind. I had to bring the kids with me."

"Okay."

"I didn't want to cancel and not come this evening. I'm getting so close to being done."

"Okay," I say again still standing at the door, taking them in. Ella has a strange look on her face, and I think she is wondering what is going on.

"Come inside," I say and move back to give them room.

"I really am sorry about this," Eric says again. He looks at me in an odd way, like he didn't think I would have cared, but now he sees that maybe I do.

Too late, we're all in this for however long he wants to work on the house.

"I made a couple of sandwiches. I can make a couple more," I say.

"Sounds good. Doesn't it, Ella?" Eric pats her on the head and tries to maneuver her around his legs, so that I can get a better look at her. She won't move. I think she's picked up on what I'm going through, and she doesn't want to show herself to me.

We all sit down at the table and eat sandwiches and drink Sprite from our paper cups. Eric does most of the talking.

"This is really good," he says taking a big bite of the sandwich.

"Glad you like it," I say.

"Has everybody had enough? Does anybody want a second sandwich?" I say, finally remembering how to be a host.

"I would," Eric's son says.

"Everett, you've had enough," Eric says.

I have to laugh. Everett is the only one saying how he feels.

"No, if he's hungry, he needs another sandwich," I say smiling at Everett and pulling out more bread from the bag.

"Everett's going to help me with the rewiring today. I'm teaching him what I know."

What about Ella? Does he want me to take care of her while their working? This is too much. I look at Eric and listen to hear what he's about to say next.

"Ella is a good girl. You can just put her in front of the Nickelodeon Channel, and she is happy."

Eric has no idea what he's asking me to do. I shouldn't have to be a babysitter for my electrician's kid. God, I can't hurt Ella's feelings, and there really is nothing else I can do. I have to give into this.

"Okay," I say glaring at Eric, leading Ella out of the chair and into the living room. He gives me this confused look, like he's saying "What?"

I turn on the T.V. and try to find Nickelodeon.

"I know the channel," Ella says and reaches for the remote in my hand.

She goes right to the channel and sits on the floor in front of the T.V.

Eric and Everett walk through the living room and make their way to the hallway and the attic stairs.

I sit down in the chair behind Ella. Strange to have a child in the house, I keep thinking. I've been trying to keep men out, and now there's not only a man, but his two children; one climbing around in the attic with his father, and the other one sitting a foot and a half in front of me watching *SpongeBob SquarePants*.

I lean back in my chair and try to relax. I'm afraid something might happen to her if I leave her in this room alone. She might disappear or something.

I watch her laugh as SpongeBob puts on a clean pair of square pants. She turns around and looks at me to see if I thought it was funny. I laugh for her sake.

"Does your brother watch this show?" I say to her.

"No, he used to, but he says he's too old now." She turns back to the T.V.

I look at the T.V., so that I can laugh with her. We sit together, watching cartoons.

She's laid her head back on the bare floor. I pull a pillow from the couch, lean down and place it under her head. She grabs the pillow with her hands and adjusts it as she turns onto her side.

She's become quiet, and I know without looking that she's asleep.

ے

I have these pictures that I took of my grandmother when I was about fourteen. She's not smiling in a single one.

The pictures were taken when I was staying over with her one weekend, like I usually did. I was nosing around in her kitchen drawers, while she was sitting at the kitchen table drinking coffee.

"What are you looking for?" she said.

"I don't know, something interesting," I said.

"Honey, the only thing you'll find in there is a pair of old glasses and receipts that I ended up not needing."

She was right; I found a pair of black-framed glasses, some green stamps, and lots and lots of receipts. I pulled everything out on the counter still searching, and then I pulled the drawer out even more. That's when I found her camera with a square flashcube sitting on top. There were smears on one of the bulbs that had already been blown.

"Hey, Grandma, I want to take your picture."

"No, Tambri. I doubt there's any film in there."

I turned the camera to the back. "Yes, there is," I sing-songed to her, and I grabbed her by the hand, pulling her up from her chair. Of course, if she really hadn't wanted her picture taken, she could have just sat there, and I couldn't have budged her one inch.

"Come on," I said.

"All right, all right," she said running her fingers through her dark hair, patting it down as she went.

"Do I look okay, Tambri?"

"Beautiful, Grandma," I said. She smiled at that as she backed up to her blue chair, finding the arm of it behind her before sitting down.

"Ah, honey, you're the beautiful one in the room."

I smiled.

"I'm ready," she said. Then the funniest thing, or not so funny thing, happened. Her face went to stone. No smile.

I stood there waiting; I think she thought I wanted to hear more about how pretty she thought I was.

"Boys are going to clamor to see you. They'll come right to your door. That's how my sister met her husband, you know."

"Okay, Grandma, smile," I said, and raised the camera to my right eye. "Smile," I said again, and pressed the button.

The flash went off, and I watched as the cube starting turning to the right.

"You didn't smile," I said to Grandma while the cube made its complete rotation. It made a swish sound as the flash scraped against the camera.

"I did, honey," she laughed while she talked. I raised the camera to my face trying to catch her laughing, but she saw me, and her face became stoic again.

"My brother Charlie was good friends with the brother of the guy that my sister ended up marrying." She put her finger to her mouth as if she was trying to get everyone straight. I wasn't really listening, and what I could hear confused me.

"One day the guy that was good friends with Charlie brought his younger brother with him. And, that's all there was to it. My sister met his younger brother, and they were married in six months time."

"You need to smile for the picture," I said sounding demanding this time.

She moved the muscles in her face as if they hurt. I didn't understand; she was always laughing, and smiling, and pretty much having a good time.

"The corners of your mouth need to go up," I said.

"I know how to smile, Tambri." She was becoming aggravated with the picture taking, the flash in her face, and me not listening to her story.

"Okay, one last time," I said smiling as I talked, hoping it would make her do the same. It did, until I clicked the shutter and then the smile disappeared. The last dead flash made the final turn on the camera.

"See, that was a good one," she said. "I could tell."

I was disgusted.

"So, you see, I know that's what going to happen with you. Somebody's just going to show up at your door," she said glad that the picture taking was over.

 ☙

I've thought about these things that have been happening in this house; these people that have descended around me. I've decided I don't know what I think. Watching cartoons with Ella the other day almost makes me feel guilty, like I'm forgetting Sammy.

I know that on the surface, if someone saw this, they wouldn't think anything about it.

"It's just a guy that needed help with his kids, and he was trying to finish up the electrical work for you," they would say.

But I know better. I know how this will go. I can see Eric looking at me, the way men do. He was testing me with the kids, wondering how I would act. Wanting to see how I would respond, how they would respond. I know he probably asked them as soon as they got in the car, "Isn't Miss Tambri nice?"

I really don't know if I am, Eric. I don't know if I can be. The thing is I know that Ella would be mine. She doesn't even know her mother, so, without a doubt she would be mine. Not like Sammy, not the same way, but she would belong to me. Am I nice enough to want that, to be her mother? Have I punished myself enough to want that for myself?

Beats the hell out of me.

☙

"I'm sorry about the other day, Tambri. Springing the kids on you and everything."

He's watching me, wanting to see my expression.

"No big deal," I say, but I can't give him any more than that. "What room are you working on today?"

"The kitchen. You want to help me with it? It goes faster when I have someone handing over the tools. All I have to do is wire each of the outlets and switches."

"Sure," I say and give him a smile.

"Fine," he says. His mood has changed. I've done that to him. He was hoping I'd say how great his kids are.

"Have you only been married the one time?" It's the only thing I could think of to fill the silence. Damn it, up until now I had avoided opening that door.

"Yeah, how about you?" he says.

And, there it is, the question I hate to answer.

I look him straight in the eye, daring him to say anything or make a funny face. "Four," I say.

"Okay," he says, and he continues to work.

"You know, Elizabeth Taylor was married eight times," I say.

"Yep, I did know that. My mom loved Elizabeth Taylor."

"Yeah?"

"Remember the last guy Elizabeth Taylor married?" Eric says, "I think he was Swedish or something. He had all this blond hair."

"Yeah, I think he was a body-builder."

"That's right. I forgot about that." He chuckles at the image of Elizabeth Taylor's last husband.

"I think Richard Burton was the one she really loved. She married him twice," I say.

"No, according to my mother it was Mike Todd that she loved."

"I hadn't thought about that."

"My mother has." We laugh.

"Yeah, makes sense. She didn't divorce him. He died in a plane crash."

I hand Eric the screwdriver that he needs, and we both turn quiet mourning Elizabeth Taylor's loss of her true love.

"Do you want something to drink while you're working, Eric?" I'm trying to make up for disappointing him earlier.

"No, I was thinking I bet we can get this kitchen done in about an hour."

"Should we time it?" I say, excited that he's turned playful.

"This is the last room to be done, you know," he says.

No, I didn't know.

He nods his head and grins.

"What?" I say.

"Let's time it, like you said."

"Okay." I look at my watch. "5:02."

"Yep, let's finish this room!" he says yelling, throwing his arm down at his side, pretending to start a race.

The game begins. It's hard not to get caught up in it.

"Tambri, I need the Phillips, please."

"Yes, sir," I say, and hand it over like a surgical nurse.

We work with precision. No playing around, no goofing off, until we realize how silly we're being and laugh.

"I still want to try to finish this in an hour."

"Me, too," I say, and hand over what he needs without him asking.

"What do we have? Three more outlets to replace?"

"Yep," I say, and we move to the outlet that I use for the toaster.

Eight minutes for each one, and now we go back and add all the switch plates.

Done, all shiny and clean.

"You know, we probably should have checked to make sure every outlet and switch worked before we put the plates on," Eric says. "Damn, I wish I'd thought of that. I think I was caught up in finishing in an hour."

He's face is falling. It reminds of my Grandmother in one of those pictures. I can't stand it.

"Let's try them all, now," I say grinning, plugging everything in to each socket. I walk over to the open panel box and move the kitchen breaker from left to right.

Eric watches, wonders what I mean, and waits.

I punch in three minutes on the microwave and press start. The sound of the heat moving inside the oven lets us know it's working.

Eric smiles at me, still unsure of what's going on. I turn on one light switch and then the other. Both come on and the room is bright.

Eric shakes his head at me like I'm crazy, and he walks across the room to the toaster, and turns it on. We both converge above it, looking for the coils to light up, and there they are, bright red, and ready to toast.

We're both close to the stove now. I turn on the exhaust, and it whirs to life. Eric hits the switch for the light above the stove, and it illuminates the black stove top. I turn on all the eyes.

I go to the pantry and pull out the blender and the mixer.

Eric takes the blender from me. He pushes the ice machine on the door of the fridge, catches a couple of pieces in his hand, and throws them in the blender. He plugs it in without bothering to find the lid. Ice flies everywhere.

"Look what you did," I say.

"So?" he says in a pretending-to-be-tough tone.

"So, this," I say and put the blades in the mixer, plug it up in the last outlet available and push the control to high. It spins, and clangs in my hand.

"What are we doing?" we both seem to be saying to each other, while we laugh, touching our stomachs, because the laughter is so hard.

I turn the mixer off, but it still feels like it's moving in my hand. The warmth of it rests in my palm.

Eric moves to the other side of the room, turning things off as he goes. The microwave, the toaster, and the two light switches I turned on. I start on my side and turn off the blender that Eric left running. We both move toward the middle of the room where the stove sets, lit by its own light, burners glowing, exhaust running. We're smiling, and catching our breath. I'm giddy from the movement and energy in the room. I know that Eric feels the same way.

The heat of the four burners reaches us. I glance over, and switch them all off. I look back at Eric, and he hasn't moved his face away from me. He smiles wider and, without shifting his gaze, turns off the exhaust, and the last light burning.

℘

Ella offers me a handful of wet dirt as we sit on the hard ground at the bottom of the bleachers. The mud spills into my palm, and I laugh as I squish it between my fingers and show her how messy I can be. She giggles and pours out the little bit of water she has left in her paper cup.

I still miss Sammy every day, but I don't listen for him all the time.

Eric sits at the top of the bleachers yelling to his son. "Stay ready, Everett. Stay ready." I twist my head towards Everett playing shortstop, and I watch him through the fence, as he bends his knees and shifts his feet back and forth.

Vickie says I'm different.

The batter hits the ball for a foul that slams back against the metal behind me and Ella. We jump and grin at each other knowing that we're safe.

I would have thought it would have been Everett, but she reminds me the most of Sammy. It may change once she's a little older, at an age he never reached. I push the sweaty hair back off of her forehead. She's determined to create a tiny mud hill in between her bare feet.

If I'd let her, she'd go barefoot all the time. Sammy was the same way.

"Strike two," the umpire yells.

Eric clutches his hands into fists, knowing that this batter hits right in the middle of second and third. Eric's coached Everett every evening for the last three weeks getting ready for this first game. Even when Everett had team practice, afterwards, they would head outside. "Okay, let's do pop ups," Eric might say. They would play until it was too dark to see the ball anymore.

Once in a while, Ella and me would sit out on the porch and watch. The horses would meander outside sometimes, too, interested in what was going on.

Eric would toss the ball up in the air and smack it with the bat. Sometimes it would worry me how hard he would hit it to Everett, but Everett would make the best plays when his father knocked it with all that he had.

Everett would yell to me and Ella when he'd make a really good play. "Did you see that, Tambri? Ella, did you see it?"

"I saw it, honey," I'd say.

"Me and Peggy saw it, too," Ella would say. She'd make sure to hold her doll above the railing so that Peggy could see.

I hear the bat make contact with the ball again, and I know it's headed towards Everett. I push myself up off the ground, and I turn and face the field. It's a high fly ball that's maybe forty feet in the air. Please catch it, Everett. He's got his glove ready, oiled palm facing up. Come on. Come on. People say, "Get it." Some shout while others whisper.

I grab for the metal of the fence with one hand. As I watch the ball spiral down towards Everett, Ella slides her hand into mine. I squeeze and her palm is gritty and warm.

Sammy squeezes back.

MAE AND MEESH

Chapter 1

Forced lessons begin with impatience and thrive on hope of distant dreams of roads heavily travelled and bent at the corners and misshaped by listeners who say they know the way and fold to the opposite of what is intended, the opposite of what is managed, the filter that binds us by circumstance and fossilized hope and determined cement attitudes of positions taken and clothes unwashed and folded haphazardly on the floor as reptiles wander the streets speaking out of turn and holding us hostage by using words that sound good, but interpreted poorly and salaciously spoken in whispers that make us bend our ears and come up for air wanting to know the secret of proper diet and mindful thinking that will instill in us the object of our desire.

Meesh lies on the couch, a couch that isn't his, awakening from the "sleeping off" of the night before. Bells ring from Eventide Baptist Church, the oldest church in town, and he listens for the silence in between, the stillness that doesn't clang and beat on his nerves.

Pulling the pink, heart-embossed cover over his chest, he winces, the material tickling his bare stomach. Lifting his head, careful not to inflict further pain, he searches the room for his t-shirt. It lays wadded, a grey heap, on top of his overturned tennis shoes, too far away for him to reach from the couch. He snuggles into the cover more.

"Mathina," he says, listening for her movements from her bedroom. She doesn't like to be called by her full name.

"Mae." The bells continue ringing. Does she go to church? He's never been here on a Sunday morning before, or any morning. He'd always hoped he would end up in her bed, but the couch is one piece of furniture closer. He smiles looking toward her half-closed bedroom door.

Proper attire is required, he thinks, as he stands up, stretching his arms toward the white ceiling hoping that the pain in his head will subside. With one long leg forward, he reaches his shirt, pulling it over his head even before he stands up straight. He adjusts his shirt, buttons the top of his jeans, and pushes his lean fingers straight back through strands of loose brown hair. He listens for Mae sounds. Still. Nothing.

A two-thirds empty gallon of milk sits on the low beige coffee table with clear, plastic cups of varying levels of alcohol cluttering the rest of the surface. Where's the vodka bottle? Meesh looks around. White Russians. Good God, who's idea was that?

He observes Mae's living room space as he sits down to put his shoes on. Sheer blue curtains hang against the long bank of windows that look out onto the street. Not many cars on this road, Meesh thinks. Black-framed photos of a teenage Mae with her mother and sisters hang in a straight line on the wall that separates the living room from the kitchen.

One of the sisters was here last night, he thinks, but which one was it? They all look so much alike. He leans into one of the pictures, staring at the siblings. There are four including Mae. Straight blonde hair and blue eyes, and none of them smile in the picture. The mother smiles, but it doesn't look real to Meesh. Nope, still can't tell which one was here, Meesh thinks.

Stale cheap beer, the only thing that Tom Fordham will drink, too good for White Russians, and putrid milk stink up the room.

It's rare that he is alone in one of her rooms. Usually, there's at least Mae, she flits and talks in quick spurts, moving in and out of herself, unsure of what or who she is. Normally though, there's always lots of people, some known, some friends of friends.

A few filled the room last night. Meesh thinks back, maybe four or five, counting him. Leaning against walls, sitting crossed-legged on the floor, tucking calves under butts on the couch. Meesh is a wall leaner, easier to watch from that position. He likes to take people in and size them up. Judge is probably too harsh a word.

The front door creaks. Meesh looks towards it, realizing that it must have been left open from last night. Who was the last asshole out, he thinks, can't even close the door. The bottom of the door sticks as he pushes hard, closing it.

The predicted rain of yesterday evening never happened, but the humidity did. Mae plugged in a little silver fan. It set on top of a beat-up yellow garden stool, but it didn't move much air around. Someone ended up opening the door. It might have made a little difference, but it seemed to make everyone happy.

"I'm trying to make it to the end of the month before I turn on the air," Mae said. The middle of her cheeks turned a faint red at the idea of having to tell everyone that things were tight.

"No problem, Mae," Meesh said, grinning at her.

They all knew anyway. That's why, most of the time, they'd end up at Mae's. She really doesn't have the money to go out, and usually someone brings extra alcohol and some snacks in case she wants something. She's the kind of person you want to do for, Meesh thinks, she's just not one to take advantage.

Most of the windows of the 1954 house had been repeatedly painted shut by the last few tenants; Meesh had offered to bring a hammer and crowbar to wedge some open for Mae a couple of weeks ago when the warm weather started. "No," she had said, "It makes me feel safer. If it's hard for me to get out, maybe it's even harder for someone to get in," she said.

The sun filters its way through the sheers removing any thoughts of rain. The morning coolness proceeds into the mugginess of the hot day ahead.

Wouldn't Mae have closed the door when she went out? Is she here? Meesh thinks. She did do some heavy drinking. Normally, she doesn't drink that much. She's usually looking out for people, patting shoulders with nervous fingers, making sure everyone is having a good time.

Meesh searches the floor for the Vodka bottle again. It might work as a mouthwash, he thinks, shit, where is it?

He uses her bathroom, observing the black and white tiles, embarrassed that Mae probably hears him peeing. He makes sure to rub a little toothpaste on his teeth and tongue before spitting it out and heading to her bedroom.

"Mae." He sings her name a little this time trying to appear playful. His head throbs more, and he gives up on the idea. He pushes her bedroom door open with his fingertips. The church bells stop.

Meesh follows the line of shadows in the room as they bend sideways over Mae. She's sprawled across the bed, still wearing her shorts and pink tank top from last night. The bottoms of her bare legs hang from the side of the bed. It looks like she fell face first into her bed, and her shoes fell right off. Meesh laughs at the thought of her being that out of it. Man, she was pretty messed up last night. Even a little drunk, she's such a jumpy, little thing, Meesh thinks.

He moves toward Mae, taking one long skinny stride, and his foot kicks the missing Vodka bottle, and the last remnants of the liquid slosh as the glass container rolls forward and under the bed.

"Shit," Meesh says in a low voice. So much for trying to be quiet. He bends down to reach under the bed and pick up the bottle knowing that when he stands back up, Mae will be pushing herself up, smiling at the thought of him making so much noise. He's grinning as he straightens up. "Sorry, Mae, I tried…"

No movement from Mae.

"Mae."

"Mae, wakeup," he says, and pulls at one of her legs.

"Jesus." He stumbles back against the door, the cold stiffness of her skin numbing the inside of his hand.

CPSIA information can be obtained at www.ICGtesting.com
Printed in the USA
LVOW10s2248300816

502552LV00015B/197/P